Debbie,
All my love,
Valerie

# BODY MESSENGERS

A Planetary Archetypal Guide for Health Patterns,
Well-Being, and Self-Healing

**VALORIE J PRAHL**

*Valorie Prahl*

**BALBOA.**PRESS
A DIVISION OF HAY HOUSE

Copyright © 2023 Valorie J Prahl.

All rights reserved. No part of this book may be used or reproduced by any means, graphic, electronic, or mechanical, including photocopying, recording, taping or by any information storage retrieval system without the written permission of the author except in the case of brief quotations embodied in critical articles and reviews.

Balboa Press books may be ordered through booksellers or by contacting:

Balboa Press
A Division of Hay House
1663 Liberty Drive
Bloomington, IN 47403
www.balboapress.com
844-682-1282

Because of the dynamic nature of the Internet, any web addresses or links contained in this book may have changed since publication and may no longer be valid. The views expressed in this work are solely those of the author and do not necessarily reflect the views of the publisher, and the publisher hereby disclaims any responsibility for them.

The author of this book does not dispense medical advice or prescribe the use of any technique as a form of treatment for physical, emotional, or medical problems without the advice of your physician, either directly or indirectly. The intent of the author is only to offer information of a general nature to help you in your quest for emotional and spiritual well-being. In the event you use any of the information in this book for yourself, which is your constitutional right, the author and the publisher assume no responsibility for your actions.

Any people depicted in stock imagery provided by Getty Images are models, and such images are being used for illustrative purposes only.
Certain stock imagery © Getty Images.

Print information available on the last page.

ISBN: 979-8-7652-4377-0 (sc)
ISBN: 979-8-7652-4379-4 (hc)
ISBN: 979-8-7652-4378-7 (e)

Library of Congress Control Number: 2023912882

Balboa Press rev. date: 07/31/2023

## NOTE TO READERS

The patients and other stories in this book are true but their names have been changed or are a combination of people so that persons are not recognizable. The exception is my grandmothers and parents who are no longer with us.

The ideas and suggestions in this book are not intended as a substitute for the individualized evaluations and advice of a qualified licensed health professional. You should consult your health professionals before adopting any of the suggestions in this book or any of the products mentioned in it. Individual differences in health or family history require individualized health assessments. The author and the publisher disclaim any liability arising directly or indirectly from the use of this book or the products mentioned in it. In addition, the statements made by the author regarding certain products represent the views and opinions of the author, and do not constitute a recommendation or endorsement of any product by the publisher.

For Aicha, Yasmina, and Apolline

# CONTENTS

Preface: Wake-Up Call ............................................................. xi

## Section One: Where it all Starts . . .

Chapter 1  In the Beginning: How Symptoms Start ................... 1
Chapter 2  Exploring Divine Feminine Resurgence ..................... 8
Chapter 3  Embracing Self-Compassion ................................... 17
Chapter 4  I Feel Like a Hot Mess: Understanding Conflicts and
            Challenges .......................................................... 19
            *Questionnaire* ....................................................... 25

## Section Two: The Planetary Archetypes

Chapter 5  Fire Archetypes ..................................................... 33
            *Mars: Courage And Self-Confidence* ..................... 35
            *Sun: Authentic Self-Expression* ............................. 46
            *Jupiter: Expansion and Soul Growth* ..................... 59

Chapter 6  Water Archetypes .................................................. 69
            *Moon: Nurturing and Reflecting* ........................... 71
            *Pluto: Metamorphosis* .......................................... 83
            *Neptune: Trust Interconnection* ............................ 94

Chapter 7  Air Archetypes .................................................... 103
            *Mercury of Gemini: Communication and Connection* ........ 105
            *Venus of Libra: Creating Sensuality and Appreciating
            Beauty* ............................................................... 115
            *Uranus: Originality, Laughter and Surprise* ......... 122

Chapter 8   Earth Archetypes............................................................ 127
             *Venus of Taurus: Home and Security, Relationships,*
             *Soul and Consciousness*....................................................... 129
             *Mercury of Virgo: Control Reactions, Release from Outcomes*....139
             *Saturn: Reducing to the Essential*........................................ 148

Chapter 9   Be Your Own Advocate and Develop a Team ................... 157
Chapter 10  A Final Fable ............................................................... 163

Appendix .......................................................................................169
Positive Strategies .........................................................................171
Endnotes ......................................................................................175
Acknowledgments ........................................................................181
About the Author .........................................................................183

# PREFACE
# WAKE-UP CALL

October 29, 1996, 3:00 a.m. was my wake-up call.

"Honey, I think the house is on fire!" I shouted frantically, shaking my husband awake. We leapt out of bed, and I breathlessly called 911.

We were enveloped in thick smoke. Panic set in.

The fire chief said it was probably breaking glass or the smoke alarm in the kitchen that woke me, because "the smell of a smoke never awakens anyone."

Firemen had pulled my husband, children, and me safely out of the house. On our ambulance ride to the hospital, I felt more grateful than ever for my life and my family, as I watched my daughter share her oxygen with Erda, our family cat.

The fire changed my life forever. I learned profound life lessons from this experience:

Stuff is just stuff. Stuff can be replaced.

People and relationships are important.

Family is important.

Life Matters. Each moment is important and precious.

Prior to the fire, I had been in a pattern of living in the past or worrying about the future, not being in the present moment. I missed many precious moments while stuck in worry or wondering what others thought of me.

I now reminded myself to be open to receiving. People wanted to help us, needed to help us. I learned to accept help with humility and gratitude rather than trying to go through it alone. I opened myself to receiving more in many ways including becoming aware of subtle energies and messages—and paying attention to what they were trying to tell me.

The greatest lesson? We are not victims in our lives.

I realized how many times I had acted like a victim and responded to life as a victim. I focused on lack and on all that was not working well in my life.

It took a major inferno to pull me out of victim mode.

Yes, that was a difficult time; and it took some time to recover and get on my feet. Fortunately, we were well insured, and our home could be repaired; yet what I learned shifted something within me and set me on a journey to discover more about myself and how I could be of service to others in more meaningful ways.

The fire was a gift in that it helped me to further shape my soul purpose. Since my life had become way out of balance, the journey to discover my true self required a continued integration, a balancing act between the visible and invisible, masculine and feminine energies, and the light and darkness within.

This book supports my soul purpose. The tools and information herein are offered to develop and enhance the integration of balance, wholeness, and self-interpretation so that others on a similar path can move forward more swiftly and easily and be inspired toward self-understanding, self-healing, and self-empowerment.

Each person is unique and beautiful; and beyond that, each physical body is an integral part of that person's consciousness. We experience everything through our bodies via our senses. Our bodies help us to interpret the world and are an expression of our consciousness. Our body's "symptoms" of illness or disease are our messengers for uncovering the magic and mystery within each of us.

We are all connected in magical ways we may not always totally understand, recognizing simple archetypal patterns associated with planets can help to illuminate common human patterns and common human experiences. Recognition of such patterns makes it possible to perceive certain life and health situations in a new light. The "messages" of these symptoms are like light switches that, when turned on, illuminate the path to self-understanding that lead to empowerment and healing. Uncovering these pathways of self-perception can enhance our vitality and even our longevity. We become aware of what needs to change and how life can be better.

Exploring some of the most frequent expressions of illness and disease in our society and in my own chiropractic practice has allowed me to identify common patterns. This helped me to better understand myself and others and to notice and recognize the imbalance of masculine and feminine energies in our society.

Exploring astrological planetary archetypes and the qualities associated with the elements: earth, air, fire, and water is a profound way to explore what the body is saying around this imbalance. In astrology, earth and water are associated with feminine energies; air and fire are associated with masculine energies. The integration of these elements and archetypes occurs deep within and is important for healing and remaining healthy.

Planetary archetypes are metaphors for the universal blueprints that affect all of us. Astrological signs—the patterns, personalities, and attributes associated with various planets of the zodiac illustrate universal archetypal patterns. The expression of archetypal patterns varies, depending on the individual's life experience and their unique genetic expression.

I use the twelve signs of the zodiac and the planets associated with those signs to describe archetypes. Physical symptoms associated with each of these astrological planets are explored later in the book. Each of the characteristics and patterns related to the planetary archetypes are represented in every person, so it doesn't matter which "sign of the zodiac" a person is born under.

The planets are used as a framework for explanation and as a template for exploration and understanding—and are not intended in any way to be used for astrological readings or to explore planetary motion. I leave that to astrology experts.

Humans have identified with the ancient wisdom of the zodiac for centuries, suggesting these archetypal patterns are universal. Study of planetary motion and the effects they have on humanity and the earth have been studied throughout history. In this book, I explore the energy of the planets; describing the characteristics of the planetary archetype using personal experience and patients' stories to illustrate patterns and characteristics. The stories are true, but in some cases I combined similar circumstances or expressions of my patients or acquaintances to protect their privacy and identity.

The location of aches and pains, and the types of illness that a person experience, can be clues to underlying problems or issues associated with a specific planetary archetypal pattern. Therefore, understanding these patterns can improve self-understanding and/or our understanding of others.

Though many other areas of study are related to archetypes, astrology, and the meaning behind symptoms, my intention is to offer perspectives which provide ways to tap into what the body is saying, and offer solutions to the messages we receive via stories and personal interpretations, and practice strategies. Interlaced are physical, emotional, spiritual, nutritional, environmental, and mental strategies to shift and improve health and well-being. I also add some guides and methodologies to provide ways to stimulate genetic pathways within the body and shift a person's archetypal energies into more positive expressions of health.

I share strategies from multiple sources including academia, research, and interviews with other physicians, therapists, and coaches. The information is for seekers, those looking to understand themselves and their physical symptoms, for students of life who desire greater understanding of health and well-being. It is for those seeking wholeness and better health. It is also for healers of any kind who walk the path with others, to provide healing insights and ideas for those whose lives they touch.

The power to create our world, our bodies, and to transform illness is in our hands. Life is a delightful, expansive, and occasionally a somewhat painful gift. The magic and mystery of this life matters. Our body holds answers if we know what and how to ask. We explore how to do the asking and provide tools to manifest a more expansive fulfilling life.

# SECTION ONE
# WHERE IT ALL STARTS...

## CHAPTER ONE

# IN THE BEGINNING: HOW SYMPTOMS START

*"The human body is the best picture of the human soul."*
—Ludwig Wittgenstein

Once upon a time, in the beginning, is where it all starts—the beginning of conflict, and the beginning of pain, suffering, and disease. The first question a healthcare provider asks: How and when did it start?

Symptoms of ill health always have a beginning, even if we are unable to recognize it immediately. I once heard a physician speaking about this say the average incubation time for a major illness can be about ten years.

Events that happen in childhood, prior to a child's ability to process and understand the related emotions, are often the beginning of emotional problems that last into and sometimes through adulthood and result in adult pain patterns.[1,2] Feelings and unexpressed emotions related to certain events can be held within the body for many years.

An individual's medical and emotional problems are not all that need to be addressed; some are issues carried in our DNA from our ancestors. For example, the children of World War II Holocaust survivors tend to suffer from a much greater incidence of depression and anxiety than the general population.[3]

Several years ago at a conference, I met Mark, a twenty-seven-year-old experiencing fear of moving forward in his life. During an extended break, we had a heartfelt conversation about his dreams and goals and how he felt unable to move to a new job or to explore new opportunities. I wanted to help, so I offered to perform an emotional clearing using neuro-emotional technique (NET), and he was very willing. NET therapy is used to help identify the root emotional and physiological causes of unexplained pain, stress, or tension that is built up over a long period, typically years, creating a pattern of responses to certain types of experiences.[4]

With such a technique, discovering a specific time or event where an emotion began is possible. By using a muscle test, the therapist notes the patient's muscle responses and answers to specific questions. Weak arm muscles in response to the questions can indicate a time frame for when an event happened and what emotions first manifested that were associated with that time or event.

When examining the specific time of Mark's causal event, I discovered that the fear emotion began during the second trimester of his time in utero. And of course he had no recollection of what that event might have been.

After the session, Mark spoke by phone with his mother, and they talked about this period in his and her life. His mother recalled a time during her pregnancy when his father had been drinking too much at a party, and she felt she had to lock herself in the bathroom with the car keys. She described the fear she experienced as. she sat alone in that bathroom, wondering what might happen next.

That flood of emotion affected her fetus, resulting in an emotional pattern change. This resulted in Mark's fear pattern twenty-seven years later. By identifying the source of a long-term pattern, Mark could now begin the healing process.

Questions remain: why does this pain, this condition, appear in the first place? What is the person's body trying to communicate? If pain and dysfunction are continually suppressed without understanding why they appeared in the first place, they will more likely return, and with greater intensity.

Physical symptoms that have been incubating deep in the body for some time represent conflicts that need and want to be addressed. Listening to the body and discovering how to bring what is unconscious into consciousness is the important first step toward healing. It is necessary to express symptoms, rather than suppress symptoms, at least initially, to uncover their message. The unconscious message is found in the body, in the symptom.

Every time someone comes into my office, they describe the discomfort and pains they feel. Everything that does not feel "normal" in the brain or body is considered a symptom. Back pain and stiffness, a throbbing headache, barky cough, wheezy chest, pounding toothache, drippy nose, stomachache, constipation, and diarrhea are all symptoms, as are depression, anxiety, and chronic irritability or "edgy" sensations. Swelling ankles, shortness of breath, high blood pressure, insomnia, or overwhelming fatigue are ways the inside of the body talks to us. Even vague feelings of discomfort, overwhelming emotions, or feelings of weakness, tingling, and numbness are symptoms. Our reactions, perhaps overreactions, to life events, are also symptoms.

The symptoms scream: *Pay attention to what is happening here!*

Even accidents are not accidents. Life sometimes requires a shake up to move forward. This has happened to me many times in my life (not just the episode with the house fire).

The typical Western approach to healthcare is to ignore these signs and symptoms, hoping they will go away. If the symptoms become too annoying, then we may head to the medicine chest and reach for a pain reliever for the headache or body ache, or an antacid for the stomach upset to suppress the symptom. At the local big box store or pharmacy, we are greeted with an enormous variety of over-the-counter medications to choose from for a multitude of symptoms. Society is taught to ignore or to muffle symptoms with medication, and we have lots of choices to do so.

When symptoms become severe enough, and fear and the inability to function creep in, it is often regarded as time to reach out to a healthcare professional trained to use their tools to suppress the patient's symptoms—not necessarily to find the deeper, underlying cause of a problem.

The pharmaceutical industry partners in this process, preferring to keep us on medications for a lifetime. The majority of Americans over age sixty-five take multiple medications to "control" symptoms. In a study of over two billion patient visits, taking more than one medication was common in 65.1 percent of the population: 16.2 percent take two or three medications; 12.1 percent take four or five medications, and 36.8 percent of us take five or more medications.[5]

Limiting the number of medications taken and looking at drug interactions and adverse effects of polypharmacy, may prevent many adverse drug reactions and hospitalizations as well as decrease the risk of falls, hip fractures, cognitive decline and other secondary issues which might have been avoided.

My mother lost forty pounds and much of her cognitive ability before it was discovered that one of the heart medications in her multiple-drug cocktail was responsible. She regained her cognitive functions when the drug was stopped, but she died a few years later after a new physician added another medication to her already-delicate balance of prescriptions.

Prescribing multiple medications is often necessary with some patients, particularly aging individuals or those with complex medical conditions; but healthcare professionals "should aim for a balance between over-prescribing and under-prescribing and consider medication appropriateness based on life-expectancy and goals of care."[6]

The question that must be asked is: why is a symptom there in the first place? Ignoring or subduing a symptom will in most cases drive the disease or condition it is "speaking for" deeper into the tissues and into the cells. This situation causes cells, tissues, and organs to react in unhealthy ways, denying their full, life-giving, life-fulfilling manifestations.

If we pay attention early and listen to what the body is trying to say with its symptoms, we can prevent debilitating problems.

> "Once you understand the difference between illness and symptom, your approach to illness becomes transformed. No longer is the symptom an enemy to resist and destroy. Instead, you discover in the symptom a partner that can help you see what you lack and overcome your illness. At that point, the symptom becomes a teacher, helping you take responsibility for the growth of your consciousness– through one that can show severity, because illness knows only one goal: to make us whole." ~Dr. Ruediger Dahlke[7]

We are often taught to quash and ignore our pain and fatigue, not to pay attention to what our bodies are trying to say. We often say, "No pain, no gain," "Put up and shut up," and "Suck it up, buttercup!" We are pushed to go to school or work unless we are "really" sick. We may be encouraged to view illness as a weakness or a lack of willpower.

My patients are no longer surprised when I ask if their hip pain is affecting their ability to move forward, or if the chronic cough is related to a communication issue. I ask these questions to stimulate connection to the messages the body is expressing, to discover deeper causes and more aggressively resolve issues.

Questioning begins the process of creating a clear intention for healthy change. A heightened emotion of fear or dread will also create change, but unfortunately results in unhealthy tissues, disease, and dysfunction. Instead of dealing with the struggles that create the symptoms in the first place, we put on a happy mask and keep plugging away, not listening to what our body is communicating. We cover our symptoms with medication and go on with our busy schedules.

"I'm fine." is the automatic response to: "How are you today?"

Often hidden behind the mask are the feelings related to issues, traumas, and conflicts in our lives. The pattern continues until there is a crisis, an illness, a breakup, a stroke, or an accident. Life won't allow us to ignore conflict or stressors forever. I was not facing some of my own symptoms and angst, with resulting consequences: witness the house fire that led to major changes in my life.

Paying attention to what our body is saying helps us see where we may be having personal yet unconscious issues. Diligently exploring symptoms and searching out their underlying meaning brings them to light where transformation occurs.

Pain sends us messages that something is not quite right. Pain is truly a gift, allowing awareness of injury and dysfunction. Medications do have a place, as do chiropractic, acupuncture, homeopathy, psychotherapy, energy healing, or other treatments or modalities used to help manage the symptoms and pains people have.

Sometimes medications are required, yet healing actually requires the active participation of the person seeking that healing. Many recognize the psychosomatic relationship between the body, mind, and spirit. Many of us know people who become physically ill when in stressful situations. Perhaps this has happened to you. However, seeking deeper insight, truly understanding patterns that have developed over time, and knowing what to do about it, will build trust in an individual's ability to prevent even the most dramatic, life-changing diseases, such as heart disease, cancer, diabetes, etc.

Listening to the body and discovering how to bring the unconscious into consciousness is an important first step toward health. We may want to express, rather than suppress symptoms, at least initially, to uncover their message. But the unconscious message is found there, in the body, in the symptom.

All the gifts are stored inside, in the unexamined recesses of our bodies. To look within can be dark and scary initially, but so worth the effort. The human body is an amazing gift of transformation that is designed to heal. Cells are torn down and replaced with new cells every day. This process is part of our glorious design, and the magical, multiple automatic processes that the body knows how to do, to keep so many cells, tissues, and organs functioning.

Healing is an ongoing process that is never-ending until we die. Yet the question remains: Why do people have these aches, pains, conflicts, traumas, and challenges, resulting in so much disease and illness, if humans are designed to heal?

The human body is an amazing gift of transformation. So what has caused our loss of wholeness, self-understanding, and self-empowerment?

History of the rise of the patriarchy tells part of the story of how society has become so out of balance. A brief exploration of history uncovers how to begin to get back to health, balance, and wholeness.

## Feel to Heal Process

Try this exercise with one of your symptoms.

- Mindfully yawn a few times, and bring yourself into the present moment. Ringing a bell, super-slow stretching, or a mindful breath can do the same thing, however the yawn is most effective.

- Identify where in your body you feel a pain or symptom.

- Describe the pain. Is it aching, pressure, burning, stabbing, throbbing, or what?

- What does this pain keep you from doing?

- How does this pain affect your life?

- Using your intuition, see how the words fit into current life situations or current conflicts. Observe if current symptoms may contain elements related to mental, emotional, or relationship challenges.

    **Example:** Mike was having neck pain at the base of the skull. The pain was tight, tender, and stabbing, affecting his motion when he turned or twisted his neck, affecting his motion and mobility and his sleep, because he couldn't get comfortable.

- Now drop the word "pain" and change it to the words, "my life situation."

- See how the words fit into current life situations or current conflicts.
    **Example:** Mike had a painful life situation.

    He revealed that he had a new supervisor at work, making his life uncomfortable. The supervisor was asking him to change the way he had been working for the previous ten years, and Mike was resistant to that change.

    He wanted to just quit and leave, but he had so many years invested in this job. He felt stuck and uncomfortable. His resistance to change was showing up as neck pain, and he felt his new supervisor was a literal "pain in the neck."

    Mike recognized that the problem was related to his own resistance to change. He decided to see me for chiropractic to get his neck unstuck physically. To keep the pain from happening again, he also decided to attend a yoga class to increase his flexibility. The benefit of the mindfulness associated with breathing in yoga helped him accept that "change is inevitable." He realized he would have to change his attitude toward this job, or get a new one.

## CHAPTER TWO
# EXPLORING DIVINE FEMININE RESURGENCE

> "Women, be more powerful with your compassion.
> Men, be more compassionate with your power."
> ~Anonymous

I spoke earlier of the need to explore the imbalance of feminine and masculine energies. One way to begin to do this is to explore the rise of patriarchal cultures. Some scholars believe that the first deity who early humanity worshiped was the Goddess, the supreme deity, the creator of all things. People later came to recognize the earth itself as feminine, and that she must be worshiped to bring forth the nourishment of the people, the fertility of the lands, as well as the fertility of the women.[7] People connected to the elements, listening to the winds, praying for water, and seeking the warmth of fire. The earth herself provided what was needed for life. Watching the movements of the sun, the moon, and the stars in the heavens signaled the seasons and the passage of time. As with all life rhythms, the pendulum swung.

Eventually, throughout Europe, the Middle East, and Asia, patriarchy and its culture of domination became the new social order. With the patriarchy came the sky gods who ruled from the heavens with absolute power. The Goddess, women, and their values were suppressed, leaving their voices unheard.

Some historians say that the total suppression of Goddess religions and the divine feminine came with monotheism in which a single male deity, all-powerful and absolute, ruled both the heavens and the earth.[8]

The monotheistic faiths were enemies of the goddess. Goddess religion was considered bad and "of the devil." All women identified with the Goddess, and her ways were also branded evil, denying women of full participation in society.

Women were subsequently considered to be the source of all evil in the world. Eve, not Adam, was the source of the wrath of God upon humanity.[9] Women were the property of men, and remain so in many places in the world. Women are not in control of their own bodies. Women have been called witches and been burned, drowned, and hanged throughout the world due to the knowledge they possess—including using natural herbal medicine to keep their families healthy. In many places, married women were (and still are), unable to own property or control their own finances.[10]

In the face of such opposition, the power of the feminine and the Goddess continued. For example, the Celtic tradition of women being able to rule equally with men, even taking lovers and leading armies into battle included Guinevere of the Arthurian legends and Boudica who, with her daughters, fought against the Romans in the first century CE.

Although the dark features of the Black Madonnas of Europe are explained by the Church as the result of either the smoke from candles in the churches, or in allegorical terms from the Song of Solomon 1:5, some anthropologists think that these paintings and sculptures are representations of the goddess.[11]

This suppression of women and of everything feminine continued through all those generations. Yet understanding the past is important for humanity to emerge from the damage of a patriarchal past and create a different reality for ourselves and for future generations. Despite the efforts of the patriarchy to crush much of the feminine or anything female-dominated or influenced, a reemergence of sorts of the female and the divine feminine has been seen since the late 1960s (at least), with the birth of the women's liberation movement across our culture, in art, music, and literature. Women's studies programs are offered in college and university curriculums, and a movement continues toward equality for women, perhaps more noted in Western society.[12] Activism is certainly present, but progress is slow, and there have been continued setbacks. The US is still without an equal rights amendment for women.

We live in a world of duality, with no escaping the opposites: in/out, up/down, light/darkness, or male/female. In early Greek philosophy, the Pythagoreans discussed the idea of Ten Fundamental Antitheses. This philosophy is about opposites (light/dark, odd/even, good/bad, left/right, male/female) and how neither extreme is ever a good thing—total light or total darkness would not be good, but a balance between the two is good, though rarely found exactly in the middle.

Wellbeing and wholeness are created by finding the balance between masculine and feminine energies within and not allowing either to dominate. Masculine and feminine archetypes have nothing to do with gender or sex. Every person has male and female aspects within.

All humans have estrogen and testosterone. To become truly whole, it is important to embrace all aspects of the self. Archetypal patterns of the divine feminine and divine masculine are expressed in the dance of hormonal components of this divine merging. Because we live in a world of duality, we have both. It is inescapable. What is called for, and will help us all, is the divine union of masculine and feminine.

A 2020 Gender-Related Attributes Study listed some of the attributes of the feminine and the masculine.[13]

**FEMININE**
Compassionate * sensitive * delicate * anxious * loving * caring * tender * warm-hearted * family-orientated * intuitive * affectionate * emotional * careful * open regarding feelings * vulnerable * sensitive * domestic * in need of affection * insecure

**MASCULINE**
Rational * analytical * strong * competitive * bold * daring * robust * confidant * career-orientated * risk-taking * pragmatic * controlling * courageous * assertive * dominant * brave * adventurous * egotistic * reckless

All these characteristics appear in men *and* women, and no single characteristic is better than another; yet the patriarchal society of the past has placed greater value on masculine characteristics.

The "sick care" industry, as I call the medical industry as it is implemented alongside the pharmaceutical industry, has roots in the patriarchy with its outside-in domination and analytical approach to healthcare. We are more likely to be told by a clinician to take a drug to treat or cover a symptom rather than for that clinician to seek out the underlying cause of the symptom in the first place. Corporate healthcare and the pharmaceutical industry are not motivated, other than by profit, to find a cure for any condition if they can find a medication to suppress the symptom, and the patient continues a drug or other treatment for a lifetime. In standard medical practice in the US, studies and research done on pharmaceuticals and other healthcare innovations have primarily been male-focused, with the needs of women largely ignored.[14]

In nature, masculine and feminine energies are balanced. Think of a seed planted in the earth. The seed is feminine, holding the creative potential to become a plant or a tree. The seed is buried in the earth, waiting for the right conditions of rain and warmth that allow the masculine energies of assertiveness and bold aggression to crack open the seed and shoot those tendrils out of the earth and into the light. This is an example of the divine union of masculine and feminine energies at work.

Unfortunately, these energies have not been in balance in our society or our bodies for a long time. The unexamined recesses of our bodies are related to our interior, the intuitive and vulnerable feminine aspects inside of the body.

Give and take, in shared masculine and feminine energies is key. "Gender is in everything; everything has its masculine and feminine principles. Gender manifests on all planes."[15]

Women were expected to suffer in silence rather than ask to have their needs or desires met. Many were not allowed to set the boundaries of their time or of their bodies. Girls were expected to be quiet and acquiesce to the men in their lives. I vividly recall my grandmother telling me I should clean my brother's room (never happened, never in a million years!). She was the oldest girl on the farm with nine children and spent her upbringing helping with the infants and cleaning up after and serving her father and brothers, washing and ironing their clothes and preparing their meals. She always valued the boys and men more than the girls in her family, and she tried to carry that tradition to her grandchildren. My grandmother was not unlike generations of women who were raised to believe women were "less than" men and should be subservient to men.

If one is not allowed to be aggressive outwardly, aggression or assertiveness must be masked to hide aggressive intent. This results in what is considered indirect, passive aggression, which I will call "female aggression." Examples of indirect aggression are spreading rumors, provocation, and inflicting reputational harm. Other ways indirect aggression shows up is excluding others from social groups and making insinuations without direct accusations. Men *and* women utilize this indirect-type of aggression. Yet traditionally it was more often women who used this type of reputational assault or provocation and for good reason.[16]

Passive aggression is when people exhibit resistance to requests or demands from family and other individuals often by procrastinating, expressing sullenness, or acting stubborn. This type of aggression can also exhibit as shutting down communication or refusing to discuss problems.

Indirect and passive aggressive behavior is a holdout from the patriarchy where women were punished for any vocal or physical aggression. They faced repercussions if aggressive and/or dominant.[17] Their aggression had to be indirect. "If I can't say what I want to say, or do what I want to do, then I am going to make life miserable for you," or "I am going to make you suffer by withholding my love and affections."

If one withholds emotions or authentic expression, their psyche is wounded, causing personal harm and not achieving the levels of intimacy that many crave. A lower amount of direct aggression is typically seen from women, which may partially explain why more women experience autoimmune type diseases as opposed to men. Women continue to be much less likely to speak up or speak out about the issues and challenges that impact their lives, so that aggression remains internal. The tendency for autoimmune disease as well as emotional patterns and reactions to trauma can pass from generation to generation in the genes.[18]

Autoimmune disease is literally a person's immune system attacking their body. Scleroderma, fibromyalgia, Lyme disease, and multiple sclerosis are examples of autoimmune-type illness. Healing from these conditions requires radical lifestyle changes.

A person with traumatized wounded feminine characteristics exhibits negative attributes such as neediness (being clingy), desperation, addiction, self-destruction, using destructive back-stabbing gossip and behaving like a victim.

A person with traumatized, wounded masculine characteristics exhibits the negative attributes of domination, detrimental conflict, violence, greed, conquest, and unhealthy competition; yet at the same time exhibits a desire to be held and/or act out to be noticed. A person may feel the need to hide their authentic nature for fear of being found out as being weak or not good enough or strong enough in some way.

Let's examine the power of the divine feminine. Accessing and embracing the divine feminine from a fresh perspective can look like: being authentic, being open to receive, and creating and honoring personal boundaries. The divine feminine requires feeling more and listening from your heart. Divine feminine power is the power of synthesis (creation), connection, belonging, and wholeness. It is the diamond emerging from the coal. Divine feminine energy is nurturing, healing, gentle, expressive, patient, and expresses emotion, vulnerability, and flexibility.

Divine feminine power requires the strength to be compassionate to the self and others. It requires the ability to be present to the moments of life, listen to the inner voices that come from intuitive feelings and insights, and heed the messages of what the physical body is expressing and feeling.

Then what about the divine masculine? What is it? The divine masculine, as opposed to being energy, is what we do—the actions we take. Divine masculine energy assertively but gently faces issues that require actions, communicates with openness and clarity, desires self-growth and understanding, is sensual, appreciates beauty, and is unique, adventurous, free, protective, and wanting everyone to feel those ways. Divine masculine energy and power include logic, reason, and action, along with adventure, strength, and courage. This divine masculine energy protects and provides. Divine masculine power radiates personal power with authenticity, seeks wisdom and knowledge, and is not fearful of being unique or original in thought or deed.

Coming to a balance of masculine and feminine within is not about making men villains but seeing how the effects of the toxic patriarchy has wounded all humanity. Women live longer than men often because of the trauma and expectations of the patriarchal society.

The patriarchal model is not good for men or women. According to an article in the *Washington Post* by Liz Plank, executive producer and host of several digital series at Vox Media, and author of *For the Love of Men: A Vision for Mindful Masculinity*, says, "Men are more likely to smoke, abuse alcohol, engage in high-risk behavior and have accidents at work. A report from the World Health Organization points to three reasons men don't live as long as women: the way men work (they endure greater exposure to physical and chemical hazards), their willingness to take risks (thanks to "male norms of risk-taking and adventure") and their discomfort with doctors (they're "less likely to visit a doctor when they are ill and, when they see a doctor, are less likely to report on the symptoms of disease or illness") . . . If men's rights activists really want to improve men's lives, then they should join feminists in dismantling bygone ideals of masculinity.[19]

In my own practice, I have often seen how men, much more frequently than women, will act as if their life or way of life is threatened before they will do anything related to improving their health. The minute the problem is gone, the patient is gone, until the next crisis arises.

Balance is created when men and women examine where they may be using too much masculine energy and not enough feminine energy and vice versa. In hindsight, some of my personal issues were associated with an imbalance in my male energy: being the doctor, primary breadwinner, boss, and business owner. The personal angst I have had to heal from was due to my primary roles in life, which are roles that have more male energy of giving out, career advancement, attempting to be in control, and being harder instead of taking in and being softer. I was great at nurturing others, but I had difficulty with receiving, nurturing myself, or allowing personal expression of the more feminine pole in the office. I felt an internal push to always do more, have more, be more; and yet I had difficulty being assertive enough to ask for what I needed or to set enough personal boundaries.

Observing and being reflective about this history of patriarchy and how it has manifested in the inner perceptions and outward expressions of life is important. Notice the patterns in your life and in your genetic heritage. Examine personal roles that are currently part of life, such as being a parent, child, employee, employer, teacher, student, leader, or member, and pay attention to the balance of energies. Are there places where being more assertive or dominant might serve? Or are there situations where being more sensitive, caring, and vulnerable would be of greater value? Look within to discover what is most important personally to create a balance of energies moving into the future.

World changes show evidence that slow change is occurring, and that balance may be possible. Mother Earth, feminine by nature, needs care and attention. Ignoring the planet can lead to our destruction and loss of life as we know it. The earth needs the divine masculine support of power through protection and action to slow down rapid changes in the global climate, as opposed to the patriarchal raping of the earth's natural resources that is our history and causes much of the damage to the planet.

Western society is slowly shifting away from traditional Western medicine to embrace more natural, holistic forms of healing. The use of complementary and alternative therapies is growing year after year. Women are stepping forward in diverse ways from politics to healthcare. Observe the MeToo movement where so many women came forward, sometimes years after experiencing sexual harassment and/or sexual assaults, and joined with others in rejecting the degradation of women that had been ignored and condoned for so long in our patriarchal culture with a dismissive attitude that "Boys will be boys." Some sexual predators, like movie producer Harvey Weinstein, received extended jail terms instead of a slap on the wrist as would have occurred even a generation before. Yet others have not yet been punished.

Historically, people who have identified as someone other than heterosexual often had to hide their authentic sexual expression due to the discrimination and intolerance of others. Gender identity is complicated, and I don't pretend to be an expert on the subject, but I honor and respect personal choice and individual expression. Male/female boundaries have become more blurred, and a range of differences have become increasingly more mainstream, as evidenced by the increase of LGBTQ characters seen on TV.[20]

Systemic racism and the patriarchal history of domination and power over others is written about and talked about increasingly, often as headline news. *The New York Times Magazine* began, "The 1619 Project," referring to the 400th anniversary of the first slave ship arriving in Virginia, in an effort to reframe the long history of people "owning" other people in

America by "placing the consequences of slavery and the contributions of black Americans in the very center of our national narrative."[21]

Similarly, "The Ransom Project" describes Haiti's history of slavery and the actual high cost they paid to finally gain independence from France.[22] Such truth telling was long overdue. Racial stereotyping of African Americans by police in Ferguson, Missouri, in 2014 triggered riots and unrest when police shot and killed a Black teenager, Michael Brown. Multiple similar incidents in other cities continued, and protests exploded across the planet when a video of the 2020 murder of George Floyd in Minneapolis by a police officer was shown around the world. The international uproar over the murder and consequent actions led to some proposed changes in legislation regarding policing in our communities. But true systemic change is slow. We have seen no reparations for a history of slavery and continued racism in the US toward African Americans or for Native Americans, who have known several centuries of abuse, genocide, violence, and attempted annihilation of their culture.

Understanding masculine and feminine patterns helps to navigate and change relationships in families, communities, and in the world. The self-empowerment of personal healing helps the world achieve wholeness since each person can only heal themselves in the dynamic, ever-changing, interconnected universe.

These patterns and expressions remind us of our connection to the elements that make up this world and the universe. Understanding and reconnecting to the feminine, which has been minimized and suppressed for generations, is necessary for the feeling of connection to earth and to water. Fire and air are related to the divine masculine principles and patterns. This background will be helpful in the exploration of the planetary archetypes and the elements they represent.

## CHAPTER THREE

# EMBRACING SELF-COMPASSION

A message that came to me years ago emerged from my consciousness and intuition rather than being something I learned in an academic environment: self-care is the greatest form of compassion a person can give to others. I recognized this in the depths of my soul, yet it has been a lifelong challenge to absorb the message and move it into action.

Self-care is the pathway of compassion for self. Compassion literally means "to suffer with," and who do we suffer with more than ourselves? When caring for others, empathy means understanding and feeling the pain or emotions of another. Self-compassion and self-empathy require acknowledging, understanding, and feeling our own pain and emotions, and doing something about it. The first Noble Truth in Buddhism is: there is suffering in the world. Each person will experience some suffering during life.

A systematic review around the meaning of the word "compassion" in healthcare provides us with this description: Compassion originates as an empathic response to suffering, as a rational process which pursues patients' well-being through specific, ethical actions directed at finding a solution to their suffering. I therefore define the term compassion to mean the sensitivity shown another in order to understand their suffering, combined with a willingness to help and to promote the well-being of that person, in order to help find a solution to their situation. This should be a duty in the daily work of healthcare professionals.[23]

Without the contrast between suffering and its opposite (not suffering, or what the Buddhists call "the beautiful state"), there would be a loss or lack of appreciation for those times of mindful awareness, being in the flow, appreciating the beauty that this world has to offer, being creative, and communicating with others.

If we are compassionate with ourselves, we will welcome the internal messages about the myriad of reasons for our suffering. That which comes from within will offer guidance. The individual then uses strength and courage to ask for what is wanted and needed, and takes the necessary actions to meet needs and relieve suffering. We have a duty to ourselves to do this. My yoga instructor calls this "fierce compassion." Gentle, soft, and reflective on the inside, and fierce and powerful on the outside, especially when it comes to setting boundaries of our time and energy.

Healing is defined as relieving suffering. Each person can only heal themselves. Others can provide tools and treatments, yet the actual healing comes from deep within the individual. We are all our own healers. Healing occurs when we have self-empathy, self-compassion, and the willingness to seek the messages from the symptoms. To be healed doesn't always mean the end of pain. But it means the end of suffering.

Often people have feelings of low self-esteem or feel unworthy of self-care. The trap can be that it is selfish to care for self or carve out time for self-care, but that thinking can and will create illness. It is too easy to stay in the victim mode, wondering what else will go wrong and questioning when the next tragic event will occur. Recurrent and spiraling thoughts drive stressful responses.

A way to understand and take responsibility for personal transformation and health is to know the kinds of issues, or combination of issues, that create the symptoms. The following chapter explores some of those issues that affect health and well-being.

## CHAPTER FOUR

# I FEEL LIKE A HOT MESS: UNDERSTANDING CONFLICTS AND CHALLENGES

> "Our own physical body possesses a wisdom which we who inhabit the body lack."
>
> ~Henry Miller

When we stay present to the conflict, issues, and challenges in our lives, we can often bravely look at them as they arrive and address them consciously. More often however, these conflicts are left abandoned, unattended, suppressed, or ignored. The conflict begins to live inside our bodies and becomes something different: an ache, some indigestion, a feeling of sadness or anxiety, or a screaming pain. Bodies talk all the time, if you just know how (or are willing) to listen.

Often these symptoms have been incubating deep in the body for some time and represent conflicts or other circumstances that need and want to be addressed. Instead of dealing with the struggles that create symptoms in the first place, a happy mask is donned, and life goes on, ignoring the messages. Life gets too busy to deal with the body or its needs. Symptoms are ignored or covered with medications, and one keeps going.

Answering "How are you today?" with "Oh, I'm fine," is a typical automatic response.

Hidden behind the façade of apparent contentment or complacency, some self-medicate with sugar, alcohol, and illicit and/or prescribed drugs to numb the feelings of dissatisfaction and frustration driving even greater discomfort. Multiple screens stop engagement with the personal psyche or with others.

Staying busy allows us to ignore what is not working, so discomfort recedes and there is no need to put in efforts to change. Self-examination or reflection requires effort, and that takes energy. Plodding along and doing what is expected is easier.

Sending conflicts, challenges, and unexamined emotions or pain inside is not listening. It is going through the motions, staying on the surface.

The word "conflict" often has a negative connotation, which is why it is somewhat easier to think of these issues as challenges. Challenges can be difficult to overcome, yet there is an inherent sense of excitement as we step into bravery, daring to face the issues and tasks put in our path. Conflicts don't have to result in a fight or in war, yet facing issues that need to be addressed requires courage and self-confidence.

Conflicts and challenges invite action, even when the outcome is unknown.

- Making a positive choice is an emboldening, assertive act.
- Increasing awareness and learning about the power within to choose a new path with better personal outcomes is empowering, energizing, and emphatic.
- Speaking up and telling others what is wanted or needed is brave and confident.
- Setting boundaries for time and energy is firm, insistent, and courageous.
- Dealing with what is not working in life, openly and despite fear, is a decided, aggressive act.

A conflict can be as simple as deciding to eat the piece of fruit rather than the donut. A challenge could be going for a walk rather than sitting in front of the computer, scrolling social media. In this case, the conflict lies in making the choice that one knows will be detrimental to health versus making the choice that adds to healthy living.

Continuing to make choices that are not good for us will result in symptoms of some kind—obesity, aches and pains, heart disease, and more.

Inflammation in the body is an example of conflict, an aggressive act. Inflammation in and of itself is not a bad thing, especially after an injury. We need the process of inflammation to stimulate healing. The body knows just what to do, and the process goes something like this: An injury or insult occurs. In a warlike way, the tearing down of tissue borders occurs as the permeability of all the tissues in an inflamed region of the body is increased. The injury to the tissues signals healing messengers to send in support.

Visualize a whole army of molecules and cells rushing to the area of injury or insult. As the tissue walls are broken down, a whole army of healing cells rush in. One can outwardly see the signs of inflammation, swelling, and redness due to increased blood flow and vasodilation of the tissues, and increased heat due to increased blood flow to the tissues.

Uncontrolled or chronic inflammation, often unseen in the physical body, causes permanent damage. Like an uncontrolled war with brutal destruction, more and more tissues are destroyed or damaged as inflammation spreads.

If one is not willing to behave with assertiveness, courage, or even aggression (if required), take actions to address situations, or speak up for self, then the body will do it by an assault with pain and chronic inflammation.

As previously discussed, tapping into feminine characteristics of listening and reflecting help us to understand the messages of the inflammation. Internal listening helps to recognize the messages in the pain or inflammation and to know what the physical body or the psyche needs or desires.

Fear, discomfort, or a busy life may keep individuals from adopting a mindful state where it is possible to do the internal listening and reflecting. It is important to stop, become mindful and present to the moment, and go into the feeling to search out the message from within.

Using a cue is helpful for many. A bell can serve as a useful reminder to take a deep breath and return to the present moment. A mindful yawn or a super-slow-motion stretch will accomplish the same thing, returning thoughts to the present moment.

Many people are separate from their body and really don't pay attention. They may only pay attention when pain is severe or impossible to ignore.

Still others think of the body as an enemy and believe pain or dysfunction is something to be destroyed or to have domination over. This is where the bell, the mindful yawn, or the super-slow-motion stretch comes in. Using these strategies means we can make conscious choices versus reacting to situations and events in our lives.

It is possible to dare to change a relationship, overcome a food addiction, or carve out time for exercise. It is possible to review the balance between doing and being. The headache, the constipation, or the elbow tendonitis may be indicating a problem or issue is not being addressed.

By stepping into the masculine power of courageous assertiveness and aggression, we support our divine feminine core and allow others to understand our individual needs and desires. With divine masculine aspects, we ask for what we want and, in turn, our needs get met.

The many types of conflicts, challenges, stressors, or traumas in our world are addressed differently depending on the type of symptom and the type of conflict. Sometimes we are not aware of a conflict, such as when we have been unknowingly exposed to pesticides or environmental toxins. Genetic variants inherited from parents are often conflicts carried to the individual. Any time we can acknowledge and address the conflicts and challenges in our lives is beneficial to our health.

## Types of conflicts, challenges, and stresses to address to lead a healthier life

*Genetic*: DNA variants inherited from parents include ancestral emotional patterns as well as tendencies for certain illnesses or diseases. Congenital anomalies are also included here.

*Chemical*: Foods eaten and supplements taken, including the types of chemicals humans are exposed to in foods and medications.

*Spiritual*: Beliefs related to the human spirit or soul, and an individual's relationship to a higher power.

*Emotional*: Reactions to the world around us: circumstances, memories, and moods, and how emotions trigger feelings and memories.

*Relational*: Our relationships with the people in our lives including the memories of early family life and how the memories of those interactions affect current relationships.

*Environmental*: Toxic home cleaning products, air fresheners, and personal care products; exposure to heavy metals; chemicals and toxins in work environments; air, soil, and water quality; plastics and pesticides; electromagnetic fields created by cell towers and computers; yeast, fungus, parasites, bacteria, and viruses.

*Physical/structural*: Physical limitations or restrictions from all causes; internal changes of structures and organs from all causes; physical motion and exercise; poor ergonomic positions at work or in front of computers along with repetitive motions that strain the body.

*Mental*: Thoughts and memories related to ideas, and opinions along with intentions, hopes, dreams, goals, and learning.

Epigenetics is the study of how our behaviors and our environments can change the way our genes function. Each one of the conflicts and challenges listed impacts genetic expression. Genes, inherited DNA, instruct the expression of every thought, every movement, and every chemical reaction in the physical body and vice versa. By changing our thoughts, choosing a different exercise program, or changing our diet, the genes affected will alter their expression. The best news is that all the conflicts and challenges involved are modifiable in some way.

No one wants to feel victim to the body, though many do. Each person desires empowerment and hope, though many have felt lousy for so long that hope fades. Realize that even small changes can have big results in the way that one feels and in how genes may express.

Any time a person blames someone else for a situation or circumstance for health problems, they are choosing to act as a victim, putting the responsibility for the condition on others rather than on the self. If you have a cold or a flu, it is not because a bug out there is waiting to attack you; it is because the immune system, our personal defense systems, are down. Anytime we have relationship problems, pieces of painful or difficult issues belong to all parties involved.

Many people are unwilling or unable to take even small actions or to change unhealthy lifelong habits. I suspect that readers of this book are probably already seekers of more expansive, healthful ways of being in the world. We can use symptoms as a pathway to personal and health transformation, and wake up to the possibility that life can be better.

We are now ready to move into the second portion of this book where we will examine the planetary archetypes and discover how understanding those archetypes greatly enhances our ability to move into a healing place, a place of self-compassion, and a place of awakening to deeper exploration into symptoms, healing, and transformation.

## QUESTIONNAIRE

This questionnaire helps to identify areas of concern or that need modification. The symptoms and memories we currently have and the genes we inherited are guidance; they illuminate the path to the next steps on the road to healing. The road is filled with hope and possibility. It is rare to have only one area of conflict.

Each of the types of conflicts and challenges previously mentioned are modifiable in some way. Review each of the categories to identify any challenges you can begin to address.

## Genetic

YES / NO I know my family history

*My family does not have a history of...*
YES / NO cancer
YES / NO heart disease
YES / NO diabetes
YES / NO addictions or alcoholism
YES / NO autoimmune or genetic disease

*I do not have...*
YES / NO addiction, ADD, ADHD, PTSD, depression, or anxiety.
YES / NO cancer, diabetes, heart disease, or autoimmune disorder.
YES / NO known genetic markers for cancer or other specific types of disease.
YES / NO recurrent health patterns, such as obesity, arthritis, or specific disease, throughout the generations in my family

## Chemical

YES / NO I eat 3–5 or more servings of fruits and veggies per day.
YES / NO I pay attention to how foods affect me and make me feel.

YES / NO I eat a wide variety of colorful foods.
YES / NO I eat a balanced diet right for me, and I don't follow fad diets.
YES / NO I prepare most of my own food.
YES / NO I buy organic whenever possible.
YES / NO I digest well with minimal bloating, belching or indigestion.
YES / NO My bowels move daily, at least.
YES / NO I read labels on foods and avoid additives and preservatives.
YES / NO I drink plenty of water.
YES / NO Water is my beverage of choice.
YES / NO I take quality nutrients to feel better or offset side effects of meds.
YES / NO I don't smoke.
YES / NO I don't take medication. (Count as 2 No answers if 3 or more meds)

## Spiritual

YES / NO My life has meaning.
YES / NO I feel as if my life has a purpose.
YES / NO I have deep beliefs related to the human spirit or soul.
YES / NO I am clear about my personal beliefs and values.
YES / NO I live life courageously and without compromise.
YES / NO I have a good understanding of my personal beliefs and/or belief in a higher power or spiritual source.
YES / NO I have a deep connection to the natural world and love spending time in nature.
YES / NO I use strategies and/or rituals to enhance my mindfulness or spiritual connection such as prayer or meditation.
YES / NO I use and trust in my intuition.

## Emotional

YES / NO I have strategies to transform or manage stress.
YES / NO I can pull myself out of a bad mood.
YES / NO I incorporate mindfulness practices.

YES / NO I can forgive easily.
YES / NO Once I understand and process, I can let go of past trauma easily.
YES / NO I am comfortable with my emotions.
YES / NO I set appropriate boundaries.
YES / NO I have an intimate relationship with a friend or a counselor with whom I can confide.
YES / NO I have someone to share my emotional ups and downs.
YES / NO I can be empathetic without taking on the problems of others.

## Relational

YES / NO I have meaningful, fulfilling relationships.
YES / NO I understand that everyone, including me has strengths and weaknesses.
YES / NO My friends can uplift me and help me to process difficult situations.
YES / NO I enjoy spending time with my family and friends.
YES / NO I trust the people closest to me.
YES / NO I share values with those close to me.
YES / NO I can disagree or have a conflict in my most important relationships and can work out differences.
YES / NO I can share my feeling with others safely and with respect.
YES / NO I experience intimacy in my life.
YES / NO I have people who are my family.
YES / NO I set appropriate boundaries with my family members and friends.
YES / NO I have memories of a happy childhood and good loving relationships with my parents.

## Environmental

YES / NO I maintain a healthy home environment.
YES / NO I have a balance between work and downtime.
YES / NO I have a healthy work environment and communicate well with coworkers and management.

YES / NO My concerns are addressed by management at work.
YES / NO I avoid chemicals and pesticides at work, at home, and in my yard.
YES / NO I use nontoxic materials and cleaners in the home.
YES / NO I avoid bleach, bleach products, and ammonia.
YES / NO I use nontoxic personal hygiene products and/or makeup.
YES / NO I take breaks from electronic devices.
YES / NO I am aware that computers and phones are electromagnetic and that I may need a protective device.

## Physical/Structural

YES / NO I exercise daily.
YES / NO I spend much of the day moving.
YES / NO I sleep well and get 7–8 hours of sleep each day.
YES / NO I utilize the care of practitioners who help with function and mobility, such as chiropractors, physical therapists, massage therapists, occupational therapists, or other physical practitioners to maintain healthy motion and function.
YES / NO I see practitioners who evaluate the internal functions and structures of my body such as medical doctors, physician assistants, nurse practitioners, functional medicine practitioners at least once per year.
YES / NO I have no physical disabilities.
YES / NO I have a physical disability; however I cope well and live my life fully.
YES / NO I am free of degenerative changes or arthritis that affect my function and mobility.
YES / NO I am free of chronic musculoskeletal aches and pains.

## Mental

YES / NO I enjoy learning new things and seek out opportunities to learn.
YES / NO I enjoy and participate in thoughtful conversations with others.
YES / NO I have a special field of study.

YES / NO I enjoy puzzles and games.
YES / NO I am free to share my thoughts and opinions.
YES / NO I keep my mind active.
YES / NO I read books and articles.
YES / NO I listen to books and/or podcasts.
YES / NO I am innovative and creative in my own way.
YES / NO I have set goals or intentions for the future.

1–2 No answers in each section (minimal concern)
3–4 No answers in each section (moderate concern)
4+ No answers in each section (areas of conflict or challenge likely require attention)

# SECTION TWO
# THE PLANETARY ARCHETYPES

## CHAPTER FIVE
# FIRE ARCHETYPES

Writing about the study of the four elements; earth, air, water, and fire began with the ancient Greeks in 450 BC. These four elements were a foundational piece of philosophy, science, and medicine for 2,000 years. Aristotle expanded the four elements to five, calling the fifth element *aether*, to describe what the stars were made of, but we have since learned that the planets and stars are made from many of the same elements as planet Earth.

Understanding some of the characteristics of the elements and how they relate to the human body remains one way to understand some of the physical manifestations of emotions and conflicts.

Fire and air express masculine energies, while water and earth express feminine energies.

Fire requires oxygen, fuel, and heat to exist. Controlled fire, like in candles, campfires, and central heating, is considered helpful. In a forest fire, wildfire, or a burning building, fires can be devastating and destructive. Air provides the oxygen, and earth provides the fuel, as in wood or fossil fuels like coal and oil. Fires can be smothered by removing the air source, cooled by adding water, or stopped by removing the fuel source.

In the body, oxygen and fuel from foods combust and create energy. Digestion itself is a fiery event except when someone's fire of digestion is depleted, and the process becomes similar to a smoky fire where the wood is damp and doesn't combust completely or burn cleanly. Fire is also represented by inflammation and pain anywhere in the body.

In work with planetary archetypes, the fire planets are Mars, the sun, and Jupiter. Astrologically and historically, each astrological sign has a ruling planet. The patterns represented are as though the planet is in its own sign. For example, Aries is the sign associated with Mars, the sun with Leo, and Jupiter with Sagittarius. Understanding those patterns can help us to recognize and understand some of our human patterns.

The planets are in constant motion and move frequently into different signs. Though it might be fun to explore how the movement of the different planets affect individuals, this is not my focus in this book. My focus is on exploring human expression and the embodied characteristics of the archetypal patterns, appreciating the feelings and the physical manifestation of the different elements and planets, and ultimately grasping the insights contained within.

Words that describe the energy of fire archetypes are: energizing, passionate, alive, dynamic, warm, courageous, radiant, expansive, creative, action, and motivational. Fire as masculine energy brings about all these positive aspects, yet due to cultural, patriarchal patterns and norms, many people (mostly women and some men) suppress their fire.

The opposite end of the spectrum can be equally temperamental, overwhelmed, destructive, brutal, overly competitive, overconfident, selfish, tyrannical, egotistic, power hungry, or grandiose if fire is out of balance. This will result in different physical manifestations depending on which archetypal pattern is represented.

I think of fire as the courageous actions we take by confronting life's challenges, and the passionate actions we take toward a fulfilling life that shift us from victim to empowered self-actualized human beings.

Courageously bring the power of fire into your life. Fire will inspire you to face your challenges and struggles and move toward joy, passion, and bliss. Like a forest fire, it burns away the old and creates new cycles in your life with power and grace. We can use fire's power to release ourselves from feelings of being a victim to events and circumstances that test our resiliency.

As I noted above, Mars, the Sun, and Jupiter are associated with the element of fire. Examining those specific planets as they relate to our bodies can bring us insight and ways to make positive change in your life.

## MARS

## COURAGE AND SELF-CONFIDENCE

### Associated Body Parts

head
muscles
joints, elbows especially
sinus
teeth and gums

### Associated Diseases/Problems

inflammation and pain of any kind
acute and chronic infections
fever
epidemics
sinusitis
allergies
upper respiratory infections
flu
tooth decay
gingivitis
periodontal disease
tendonitis, especially elbows
muscle and joint pain
headache
migraine

Conflict and inflammation have to do with the element of fire and the astrological archetype of Mars, the planet closest to the sun and the god of war. This male energy is related to power and aggression. Elbows, hands, and teeth also relate to Mars energy. "I can't handle it," "I elbowed my way in," or "I bit off more than I can chew," are examples of our culture's way of expressing conflicts related to Mars.

Much of what I covered in the previous chapter, describing different types of conflict and associated inflammation, has roots in Mars energy. Mars energy is related to the conflicts and challenges in our lives and the courage and self-confidence required to overcome and transform the conflicts so that illness is not expressed.

Dawn, a friend and patient, had an important meeting on Saturday. She knew she had to be there. She was part of the planning committee, and there was no way she was going to miss the event.

The day before the meeting, she had sinus pressure and body aches. Her face hurt, and her eyes watered. She felt a nagging throb under each temple. What was she going to do?

She made the decision that the symptoms would not keep her from her obligations. She wasn't going to panic or stress about it. She would be fine and wasn't going to miss the event.

In her daily meditation, she went silent and asked for guidance for what she needed to heal. Dawn is keenly aware of what her body needs, because she pays attention to it. She has learned that her body is not separate from other circumstances. Her symptoms are not enemies to be destroyed, but her partners and friends.

Just as she would ask one of her clients what more she could do for them, she asked her body the same question. *What is it that you need?*

She rested and drank warm herbal tea and water most of the day. She canceled a couple of phone meetings, and she took some extra vitamin C and zinc. Dawn uses essential oils, and she used the ones that would boost and support her immunity. She took a nap and went to bed early. She woke up the next morning clear and bright and ready for her big event.

The power of the mind and the body work together. Immunity can be boosted or depressed powerfully with our thoughts. This is the power of epigenetics. When we combine our thoughts with the right actions, most viruses and bacteria do not stand a chance.

We all have viruses and bacteria living in our body at any one time. But only when we get out of balance can colds and flu bugs take advantage. If our stress is running the show, we get out of balance easily, and our immunity is stifled.

When I was going to chiropractic college, I had a cold every three months when final exams rolled around. I swear I never had enough tissues! (It was hard to focus on a correct answer when my nose was dripping and I ran out of tissues.) My children were both under age five at that time. I was constantly exhausted and overwhelmed. I studied late into the night and had to be in class by 7:45 a.m., after dropping off the kids at daycare. My poor immune system didn't stand a chance.

Stress is the major "down regulator" or suppressor of immune response. My body had gotten into the habit of stress. I could head into fight/flight just thinking about the next quiz or exam. I wasn't listening to my body or asking my body what it needed. I also had a very difficult time speaking up for myself or being assertive or aggressive in any way. I was painfully shy from early childhood, even having difficulty raising my hand in class to ask questions. My mother kept threatening to take me to assertiveness training.

In chiropractic college, I kept busy dealing with toddlers, diapers, and daycare, while in a constant state of worry, fatigue, and stress, as I studied late into the night. No wonder I had so many colds; and some days I wonder how I survived!

Those were the years my hair turned significantly whiter. I was probably 50 percent white by the time I graduated from chiropractic college and turned thirty. It has taken me a lifetime to be aware and overcome that habit of stress and learn to be more aggressive in healthful ways.

## Strategies

My genetics indicate that I have a tendency toward shyness and introversion, but I have learned to compensate for that tendency. Now I can speak up for myself, speak to a group, and reach out to strangers. I still see my shyness and fear of speaking rear its ugly head occasionally, especially when I am tired or haven't spent enough time alone to regroup and refresh.

Every major disease has its roots in an altered stress response. This includes, but is not limited to, heart disease, cancer, diabetes, and lung disease—the major causes of death.[24] This is what I tell my patients now if they want to boost immunity: "Get the stress habit turned down!"

Stress is a habit, and the best habit to get personal control over. Begin to have awareness of the times when autopilot takes over, spiraling into stress reactions, anxiety, and "overwhelm." Stress response is a physiological event, a cascade of stress hormones flooding the body. The body senses danger of some kind, stimulating the cortisol-releasing factor from the pituitary gland in the brain. This sends a message to the adrenal gland to release cortisol and adrenaline into the blood. Increased cortisol stimulates the release of glucose, sending fuel to the brain and muscles. This is the fight/flight response that gives us the ability to run away from the tiger. Important in the past for the survival of our species.

Unfortunately, in a busy world, the tiger lives with us, at least it feels that way, resulting in many having increased cortisol levels much too often. These increased cortisol levels and associated increased blood sugars stimulate the release of insulin. Insulin's role is to move those sugars into cells, so the glucose can be used as fuel. Too much circulating insulin from too frequent stress causes increased inflammation and increased fat storage.

If cortisol is increased at night, it will adversely affect sleep. If stress reactions are chronic, the adrenal gland decreases its ability to replenish cortisol, and the person completely runs out of steam and can no longer adapt to the world. They are overwhelmed.

Stress reactions can be such a habit that the stress hormones can be released just at the thought of impending danger, and that type of thought has been linked to chronic pain. Awareness is key to changing the cascade of events.

It is too easy to let stress go into autopilot and run the show. Emotions are just chemical reactions in your brain. Emotions are to be observed and examined. Humans can always choose a different road.

People often say; "I am stressed," or "I am sad." No feeling is who or what we are. Be the observer of the feeling. Step back from it and watch yourself experiencing the feeling. Be aware of the memories that are triggered by the feeling. Be grateful for the ability to feel, and for the guidance that the feeling is providing.

Over time, you can catch yourself more quickly and choose different responses. Use reflection and contemplation (feminine aspects) before acting. When you speak and act from anger, fear, or frustration before you sort out and reflect on what the emotion is showing you, that communication (our outward male expression) is more likely to break down or be ineffective.

Harsh words spewed in anger at another person rarely improve communication or connection. Incredibly important, however, is to let others know your feelings. It is important to feel heard. Wait to communicate until you have time to sort out the emotions and can express your feelings more clearly. Wait until you are able to *respond* and not merely *react* to the emotions.

Another strategy I found helpful to check the autopilot reactions and separate my authentic observer self from stress and stressful emotions is to name my emotions. I learned this from the book, *The Dark Side of the Light Chasers* by Debbie Ford.[25] When Angry Ala, Pitiful Patty, or Resentful Rhona show up, I can acknowledge them, my named emotions, and remind them that they are not driving the bus of my life! Valorie Victim is welcome to come along for the ride, but she is not going to drive! The part of me observing my emotions is who drives the bus.

I do not want to totally dismiss the information a negative or stressful emotion is giving me. I know it is there for a reason. If I ignore it, pretend it doesn't exist, or cover it up, I send it in deeper. It is there to give me guidance to know this is not the road I want to be driving on, or the path I want to take. I get to choose a different road and a different response.

We want to embrace the feelings and emotions that enhance life and joyful experience. This sometimes means shifting the focus from the painful emotions swimming around in the head and heart, and finding one small thing to feel good about. This changes the focus to give a new uplifting perspective. You might observe a flower's fragrance, listen to music that stirs your heart, or dance around the kitchen. Scientific evidence shows that focusing on pleasure and pleasant events can interrupt the formation and integration of negative memories in the brain.[26]

Taking a nap is an effective pattern interrupt; drink in the warm comfort of the pillow and how good the soft blanket feels about you. I find it helps to have a long list of positive strategies to draw on to shift into a more positive state. A list of suggestions and guidance is found in Appendix A.

Be aggressive in developing personal strategies to bring down stress and anxiety. Here are a few proven ways to alter a stressful body response:

- Mindfulness
- Exercise

- Meditation
- Prayer
- Massage
- Hugs
- Yawning

After our house fire, we asked for help from friends to supply us with clothes until we could buy more. We had friends with helping hands to sort through the debris, and listening ears to help us process the trauma.

Always try to reach out to others to ask for the support you need. Search out all the ways to walk a new path. Find a counselor or coach who can support healthful change. I have worked with several coaches and counselors over the years, and I can say with confidence that I have learned from each one.

If stress is a big deal, and a habit that results in stuck stressful patterns, utilize as many strategies as possible and put together a team of support. Knowing just what to do to shift a stressful response and knowing we are being supported builds self-confidence. Aggressively taking actions to search out good foods and eat healthfully, along with taking compassionate care of yourself, is powerful and courageous.

In the body, stress is stress. An emotional event like waking in a panic because you are late for an appointment; or a chemical stress, like drinking too many caffeinated beverages or eating too many cookies, will result in the same physiological stress response with the flood of cortisol, blood sugar, and insulin. Because the body cannot tell the difference, and it will respond the same to any stressor.

Limit the sugar, caffeine, and processed foods because they use up the nutrients required to physically deal with stressful situations. Eating poorly results in a double whammy, as these foods decrease your ability to respond to life's stressful situations. Find a practitioner who can recommend the right nutrients to support you. Lots of nutrients promote a healthier stress response, however the need depends on the individual. A functional medicine doctor might need to look at cortisol levels at different times of the day to determine an appropriate plan.

In my practice, I utilize a salivary cortisol test to decide on the correct nutrients to recommend. Taking appropriate nutrients to stay healthy, support stress handling, and support the immune system is an aggressive positive act.

## Nutritional Strategies

With so much confusion about what nutrients a person should take to boost immunity, it can be baffling to sort out. Here are some of the big players:

Vitamin D3 is likely the biggest player in immune function, and it can also modulate pain. Most people in the northern hemisphere go months without the ability to expose our skin to the sun and need to take additional vitamin D3 to have adequate immune function. The "normal" range is 30–100 ng/ml on a blood test, yet 30 is not enough for adequate function for most individuals. I recommend supplementing with 5,000 iu (1,500 mcg) per day in the winter, and 2,000 iu (600 mcg) per day in the summer until your blood tests show ranges of 70–100 ng/ml; but these amounts vary with different individuals. Deficiencies occur because most of us don't hang out under the sun with 60 percent of our skin exposed, and many with sensitive skin, like me, burn easily.

Vitamin D is actually a hormone in the body, because you can make your own from your skin, and it works right along with all your other hormones. D is also found in more than 700 different enzymes. All the hormones dance together and support each other. I have found many people with adrenal gland issues, thyroid dysfunction, pancreatic problems, and even digestive problems improved when extra vitamin D was added.

Some individuals need vitamin A or vitamin K2 to get the vitamin D3 to work, due to certain genetic variants. The VDR single nucleotide polymorphism is the technical name for the primary genetic marker for immune system function. If the VDR works well, it signals the immune system to work, fighting infections with T-cells and macrophages. If unsure whether this genetic pathway is an issue, consider taking D3 with vitamin K, because K helps to signal minerals where to go in the body.

Vitamin D3 also works synergistically with calcium and magnesium in the body. Vitamin D3 and K are both important for absorption and signaling to the minerals what tissues need the support.

In addition to immunity, vitamin D3 pathways in the body play a role in preventing autoimmune disease, depression, joint pain, cravings, and addictions. Many diabetics are D3 deficient.[27]

Vitamin D3 also affects cardiac function, brain function, and bone density. Every single cell in the human body has a vitamin D3 receptor, an indication of how important it is.

If you have never had a baseline vitamin D test, I recommend it. Pay attention to what time of the year the baseline reading is done, especially if you live in the northern US or northern Europe where sunlight is scarce in winter.

Vitamin D3 is not easily available from foods. Fatty fish, like mackerel and salmon, have some vitamin D, as do eggs and beef or pork liver. Some foods are "fortified" with vitamin D; however, the vitamin D added to dairy and soy milk is primarily vitamin D2, which is not as bioavailable (absorbable). Vitamin D3 is the most absorbable form.

Since vitamin D is a fat-soluble vitamin, which means fat is required to absorb it, vitamin D is best taken along with a meal that includes fat. I recommend that patients take vitamin D with a larger meal more likely to have fat.

A person with a missing gallbladder or gallbladder problems may have trouble breaking down fats and may require additional nutrients or enzymes to get vitamin D or any fat-soluble vitamin to absorb when taken orally. Talk with a nutritionist or functional medicine doctor if your vitamin D levels don't reach optimal levels. The "normal" range on a blood test is 30–100 ng/mL, however the optimal level is closer to 60–70 nl/mL.

Why is vitamin D such a big deal now?

- Our society has become sun phobic due to fear of skin cancer.
- There are minimal amounts of K2 in the environment.
- People had access to more cod-liver oil in the past.
- Low-fat diets were recommended for a number of years.

## Vitamin C, Zinc, and Selenium

Vitamin C, zinc, and selenium are antioxidants that augment immune function. So do the colors, the reds, purples, orange, green and yellow phytonutrients found in foods.

NAC, or n-acetyl-cysteine, is a precursor to the body's most potent antioxidant, glutathione. Glutathione prevents damage to cells caused by free radicals, peroxides, lipid peroxides, and heavy metals. Glutathione is available to buy, but it is quite costly and difficult for some to absorb. NAC is easily absorbed and also stimulates lymphatic motion and circulation, so it supports kidney and liver function and helps people with respiratory conditions. In addition, it can help to stabilize blood sugar, help with brain function, and reduce heart disease risk.

Each person is unique and has unique needs. Seek the help and support of someone who understands natural immune boosters when recurrent infections occur. There are appropriate times for antibiotics, yet they should be used sparingly, rather than a first line of defense.

Don't bother taking probiotics while taking an antibiotic. Since antibiotics kill both "good" and "bad" bugs, it is just a waste of money. There may be exceptions, but save the probiotics until the antibiotics are gone; then hit them hard, double the recommended dosage for a few days!

## Creative Visualization

Flame exercise: Close your eyes and visualize a problem, concern, or any conflict as a flame sitting in front of your third eye in the middle of your forehead. Observe the flame in your mind's eye; as you take a deep inhalation, draw that flame into the middle of your brain. Staying mindful, ask your brain to resolve this problem in the best way possible. Listen for intuitive messages to hear solutions and best strategies.

## Emotional Strategy

Allow yourself to feel anger, frustration, sadness, fear, shame, or other emotion. Emotions are meant to be felt and experienced, allow yourself to feel. The emotion is not you, it is a chemical physiological event. The emotion is guidance. Is this emotion something to move toward and create memories of, or is it simply information to be noticed, transformed, or released?

## Relationship Strategies

The best way to improve relationships with others is to maintain a healthy, happy relationship with yourself. The more time spent using the strategies and improving the areas of self-growth, the better are your relationships.

You cannot expect anyone to fix you but you. True love emerges when you are willing to love and to care for yourself. We are each our own best guru.

Issues and conflicts with coworkers, parents, siblings, or partners are inevitable, and it is important to be able to express feelings and to open or keep open channels of communication. Heated arguments are not effective, however being able to express anger, frustrations, and a whole range of emotions is vital in healthy relationships.

Pick the right battles with others. Remember Wayne Dyer's question, "Do you want to be right, or do you want peace?"

## Mental Strategies

Spend time reflecting on the values that mean the most to you. Get really clear on what those values are. Getting clear on values can be life-enhancing. People who live in congruence with their values lead longer, healthier, and happier lives. Having goals and dreams and courageously taking actions and moving toward them leads to a joyous and more rewarding life. Decide what it is that would be personally fulfilling and would bring you closer to the values that mean the most to you.

## Environmental Strategy

Avoid food additives. Read labels to limit the number of food additives and flavor enhancers in your foods. No one is deficient in food colorings! Have awareness of these added colors, along with added chemicals and flavor enhancers that stimulate appetite in foods. Be aware that chemicals to keep food appearing fresh are often used in buffet tables. Many people are sensitive to additives like monosodium glutamate (MSG), which can have neurotoxic effects for many. MSG has many other names including natural flavors or flavor enhancers.[28]

## Physical Strategies

A yearly blood workup and an annual physical is appropriate. If blood levels are out of range, look at what blood levels are indicating, and see what can be changed with healthy life changes prior to treating with medications. Dental checks and cleanings also help to prevent health issues. Take time to chew food thoroughly. Dental health and gum health can be indicators of other health issues, including heart disease.

## Thoughts have power!

Remember epigenetics? This is the epigenetic connection. A person is born with genetic markers related to immunity and inflammation and adding nutrients can help with immunity and inflammation; however, if there's a belief that a cold will occur every spring, or each time the grandchildren come to visit, that reality will be created. If one is certain without an early flu shot, the next flu might kill, that reality is created too!

Thought patterns are inherited just like skin color or a tendency toward heart disease. Observe the words of the elders in your life or in your memory. Are they the victims of life, pain, and suffering? Do they focus on everything that no longer works? What patterns and words do you recall? See what pain and stressors they had to live with. It is said that trauma and emotional patterns can be carried through seven generations. We have the power to change the pattern.

Take a second look at Dawn's example. Stop, listen, and ask the body what it needs. What stressors need to be addressed? What has become embodied? The body wants to be heard. What can be done aggressively and bravely to address and deal with the situations and stressors in life? How can you use your courage and self-confidence to do just that? Trust in the body's innate, inborn, ability to heal and to maintain health.

## SUN

## AUTHENTIC SELF-EXPRESSION

### Associated Body Parts

    heart
    circulatory system
    eyes

### Associated Symptoms and Diseases

    heart disease
    congestive heart failure
    atrial fibrillation
    hypertension
    abnormal heart rhythms
    aorta disease
    pericarditis and other pericardial disease
    Marfan syndrome
    congenital heart disease
    coronary artery disease (narrowing of the arteries)
    deep vein thrombosis and pulmonary embolism
    myocardial infarction/heart attack.
    heart muscle disease/cardiomyopathy
    pericardial disease
    refractive errors
    age-related macular degeneration
    cataract
    diabetic retinopathy
    glaucoma
    amblyopia
    strabismus

After about fifteen years, I felt a lot of frustration with my chiropractic practice. I was expected to follow a specific rhythm, living by the appointment book, with obligations to patients, staff, overhead, and mortgages.

People came in year after year with the same problems. I had begun to feel as if I was a Band-Aid, Band-aiding recurrent problems and not fixing them.

I always had a great interest in nutrition and nutritional supplementation, so I traveled all over the country, taking classes on nutrition. I swore I would never look at biochemistry again after leaving college. I was mistaken. Studying nutrition helped to see chemical and physiological pathways in the body in a new way, and opened the doors to greater understanding.

I received my certification in clinical nutrition and began recommending specific nutrients and designing nutrition programs for my patients. It made a huge difference in the lives of many of my patients. I thought I had found my Holy Grail, the answer to fix any willing patient's problem: I just had to add in the right nutrients!

The functional medicine strategies, combined with dynamic muscle testing I utilized in practice, helped people with the recurrent issues such as chronic digestive issues, muscle aches and pains, headaches, sleep issues, stress, fibromyalgia, and menopause symptoms.

I continue to this day to make nutritional recommendations, yet then as now there were patients with problems that were not going away and not responding to my recommendations. I couldn't fix them, and I couldn't figure out why; and I felt somehow personally responsible.

My quest led me to classes in emotional-release techniques, to uncover, identify, and release "stuck" emotional patterns held in the body. Once again, I got great results helping patients shift emotional patterns in a safe noninvasive way.

Yet patients were still resistant to making the necessary lifestyle and dietary changes necessary to see improvement. I learned a lot, I knew how to guide people, but there were still gaps.

I believed something was wrong with me. Why couldn't I figure it out? Where was that resistance coming from?

All the while, I was gaining weight, my joints were sore, my digestion disturbed, and I frequently felt down, depressed, tired, and frustrated with life and my business. I was in debt. I felt lonely.

When away from the office, I walked along the path, watching the water of the Cedar River flow as my own tears flowed down my cheeks. I dreaded going to the office. I had wonderful staff but, as a perfectionist, I could only focus on the things they did wrong. My hands hurt when I was working on my patients. My life revolved around the appointment book. I was the doctor, the boss, and the business owner who had to keep it together and pay the bills. Put on a smile and keep going because "You have responsibilities, Doctor!" There was no ease, no balance, and no flow except for the tears down my cheeks. I allowed myself to feel the victim.

It was around this time that we had the house fire.

The people who were drawn to me just wanted relief, because that is what I wanted. I wanted a magic wand to make everything better. I escaped from my feelings as I sipped on wine and ate chocolate. I wanted to run away from responsibilities. I wanted to be like the heroine in my favorite movies who were women being rescued with money and love. I was already working so hard, how could I do more?

In hindsight, my angst was due to my primary roles in life, which were associated with male energy, being the doctor, primary breadwinner, boss, and business owner. These roles have more male energy of giving out, being harder instead of taking in and being softer. I had difficulty with receiving, being softer, allowing personal expression of my more feminine pole. I felt a push to always do more, have more, be more.

Resistant to facing my own conflicts and difficulty with authenticity, I put on a doctor mask each morning on the way to the office. The people in my life, my personal mirror, are those who also had resistance to making change and facing their own conflicts. I didn't understand the concept of projection at the time, so I was unable to see what was occurring.

Projection is defined as the mental process by which people attribute to others what is going on in their own minds. The resistance to making changes had been in me all along, and I wasn't able to perceive my own resistance.

I made a lot of mistakes. I sold my very busy, lucrative practice and moved with my husband to a small town near to where we had a lake home. He knew I was unhappy, but he didn't know how to help me.

I started a new practice and soon realized that I had created a bigger mess. I was running away from my feelings and, instead of making life better, I was now strapped for cash, feeling even more frustrated and lonely.

People came, but I had not done my due diligence when I ran away to realize that this smaller community meant a much smaller practice. I just wanted to get away, and my ego was telling me that it was the right decision. I created the same chaos, the same feelings, but with much less money!

So many wait for a crisis before being willing to look at what needs to be changed. I know I did. I experienced one crisis after the other and stayed constantly, chronically stressed.

I was floundering, so I read, studied, searched, and learned. I kept the small practice open in that small town so I could have at least some money coming in.

I spent snowy winter days watching the chickadees, tufted titmouse, nuthatches, and downy woodpeckers as they flitted from the bushes and trees to my bird feeders on the deck. I watched out the window to the lake below as eagles flew high over the lake on their way to the dam where the water was open for fishing. The water held its power even in its frozen splendor.

In the summer, on my days off and in the early morning, I strolled along our meadow path, picking gallons of black raspberries and blackberries, or got my hands in the soil while weeding in the garden, since we grew most of our own food. It was a time of deep connection to the healing energy of mother earth.

I sat and meditated on a downed tree while the bees buzzed around; and as I meandered back home, I spotted where the deer had lain the night before. Birds, bees, and butterflies filled the air and sang their songs as they danced from wildflowers to tall grasses waving in the breeze. I saw the deer each day and watched coyotes lope across the meadow in the distance.

As often I could, my journeys took me to nearby forest paths. Ancient trees, big-horned owls, and the soft forest floor offered a haven and a connection between my soul and the earth. My soul needed this time and this place, connected to nature, to discover what it was that I wanted.

Eventually, we sold our lake home, sold my small part-time practice, moved to a new community, and I started a third practice, working along with one of my long-time colleagues. It wasn't a perfect solution, but it was steady money, and I had healed enough to get back into full-time practice. I had thought about and tried a few other avenues to make money, but they didn't pan out. It was not meant to be. I still felt lost, yearning for something different and with greater fulfillment. At least I didn't have to run the practice or worry about paying the employees or shoveling snow in the winter. I just had to show up and care for people.

I continued my healing journey, the journey of my heart.

I took a course in shamanism, a practice of divination and healing. It was a reminder that healing doesn't come from me. Healing energy comes through me. I am not responsible for the healing of others. I began to release myself from the expectations that I had put on myself as "the doctor" and let myself be "the healer," a conduit for healing.

The shamanic classes reminded me to allow healing to be a sacred experience and to release from outcomes. I realized that too often I had taken on the responsibility of the outcomes, and it was wearing me out! It was not my job to heal anyone! Each person heals themselves, and that healing energy comes from above-down-inside-out. This is the chiropractic philosophy I first learned from my years at Palmer College of Chiropractic. I am just a conduit. I needed the reminder.

I have incorporated ritual practices as reminders to listen and allow guidance; some would say intuition, into my work with people. This is as simple as asking for divine guidance to come through and to support me in my care of others.

It was at that time that I took a course and learned about the universal archetypal patterns that can create heart disease, cancer, diabetes, autoimmune, fibromyalgia, lung disease, thyroid, and more.

I share my story here because it has taken me a lifetime to step into my authentic self, to release from the masks and the multiple roles that I play(ed) and to express myself more fully in the world. I have genetic and ancestral history of heart disease from my father as well as my mother's line; and when I reviewed my own genetic information, I recognized how it could easily express itself within me.

I continue to incorporate all I have learned into my own life and continue to work on my own resistance to healing. It is still there, but I am making progress.

I use an integrative approach to assist my patients to heal pain and dysfunction and deal with the stresses and conflicts that may keep them from moving toward the life that they long to live. I have also learned to set more boundaries. I take more time for self-care, and I no longer feel as if I am putting on a mask prior to seeing patients.

Hal, a patient of mine, was walking across the parking lot of the building supply store to his Ford F150 when he felt some tightness in his chest. Just fifty-six, he thought it was his childhood asthma flaring up since he had noticed some breathlessness while doing his carpentry work over the past week. It passed quickly, so he ignored it. Later that day when sitting down to dinner with his wife Susan, it happened again.

Susan was frightened by the episode, even though Hal said it was no big deal. She knew Hal had not been in for a physical for at least eight years, and this time she insisted. She observed his habits and knew something could be seriously wrong. He had been putting on weight, drinking too much beer, and grabbing lunch from local convenience stores while working on the multiple construction projects he was forever trying to balance.

The doctors ran a battery of tests and soon discovered that he had blockages in multiple vessels of his heart and was going to require a quadruple bypass. Surgery was scheduled immediately.

Hal decided at that very moment when the doctor told him that surgery was imminent that he was not going to let his heart slow him down. He and Susan had goals and dreams, plans to travel to Paris to see the Eiffel Tower and to wander the streets of Paris. He loved Susan so much, he wasn't going to let her down. Besides, his favorite wine was French, and he wanted to share a glass with Susan where it was grown.

Following the surgery, Hal began cardiac rehab. He exercised and realized just how out of condition he was. He worked really hard to strengthen and heal.

The hospital provided healthy eating courses, and he and Susan both attended. They learned ways to eat more healthfully. They adopted a Mediterranean diet with lots of fresh ocean fish and vegetables. They sought out my advice on what nutrients to take to prevent further problems and to counteract some of the adverse effects of the medications he was now taking.

One year later, Hal was enjoying a rare glass of his favorite French wine as he and Susan were celebrating. "Susan," he said, "let's get on a plane this time next year and celebrate our fortieth anniversary in France."

Plans were set and the two set their sights on the trip together. Hal continued his cardio and strengthening exercises.

The two had a delightful trip, taking a boat trip through the French countryside and having multiple excursions through dazzling cathedrals, museums, and castles. They hiked for miles and climbed hundreds of steep steps; then on to Bordeaux where Hal rejoiced as he accomplished his goal of making it to the winery where his favorite wine was produced. His heart was full as he held Susan in his arms, and they looked out at the vineyard and its magnificent views together.

Hal's story illustrates his desire to live his life to the fullest and to express his love.

Just as the sun is the center of the solar system, the heart is the center of our body. In traditional Indian medicine and philosophy, using the seven energy centers called chakras, the heart chakra is the center one. There are three above and three below. The three upper chakras, in Indian tradition, connect us to the energies of the heavens. The three lower chakras connect us to the energies of the earth. The heart chakra is the blending point, the sacred center, the point between the heavens and the earth.

Even though the heart is listed under the male aspect of fire doesn't mean it is without female aspects as well. The heart is enveloped in the pericardium, a protective enveloping membrane, that by its very nature is feminine because it nurtures and protects the heart. The four chambers of the heart allow for the influx of blood, the feminine aspect, as well as the pumping out of the blood, the male aspect.

When speaking of love and connection, most don't reach for the head; the touch is to the heart.

Heart disease is the leading cause of death. If the held belief is that exercise, taking statins, and hoping for the best is going to prevent heart disease, one is sadly mistaken.

The human heart beats nearly 3,000,000,000 times in a lifetime. It has enough force to circulate blood through over 100,000 miles of vessels. It's pumping power could empty an Olympic-size swimming pool in a week. It is self-sustaining and even feeds itself. Wow, what a powerful organ! It is easy to forget how very precious it is.[29]

In the heart/brain connection, the heart appears to have its own intelligence from which the heart sends messages to the brain—even the higher centers of the brain. The brain responds with either feel-good chemicals, like serotonin and endorphins, or with chemicals that promote stress hormone release, such as cortisol-releasing hormones, within the body.

Listen to the messages from the heart. Ask your heart what it needs or what it is saying. It is not enough to just be logical and be in the head. Take the heart's desire seriously. Do you seek adventure? Or is it your mission to be of service in some way? What are the burning desires that will express your authentic self? Truly take things to heart.

If there is a family history of heart disease, now is the time to start listening to the heart. Don't wait until heart disease manifests, by then it may be too late.

The heart has its own electrical system that triggers the heartbeat. This system is measured on an ECG/EKG test. The heart rate measures how many heartbeats per minute. The heart rhythm is the coordinated pumping action of all four heart chambers, which is signaled by this electrical system.

Our hearts want us to find our personal rhythm and balance, not a rhythm imposed on us by others. It means singing and dancing to our own tunes and following our heart's desire with courage and bravery.

It is easy to be hard on the self, forcing the brain and body to follow specific rhythms that leave no room for ease and flow. These rhythms can be imposed on us by others or by self-imposed obligation.

## Nutritional Strategies

The heart requires a lot of nutrients to keep it functioning for a lifetime. There are multiple systems in the body to review and to decide what is best for the heart. I look to requirements of the muscular system to figure out what the muscle of the heart requires. The heart needs adequate protein broken into amino acids to build new heart cells.

The heart cells and all muscle cells have the most mitochondria, the "powerhouses" in their cells. These tiny organelles, the mitochondria, make energy. This is vitally important, the essence of life since life depends on energy! An organism that cannot make energy dies.

The process of making energy requires multiple nutrients and multiple steps. Too many to discuss here, yet let's look at some modifiable factors and the heart's primary players.

Coenzyme Q10 is important for making energy. The body makes it. Unfortunately, many medications interfere with CoQ10 production and function. Cholesterol-lowering medications and some diabetes medications impact the body's ability to make CoQ10. This is why so many people have the side effect of muscle aches and pains when they take statins, as the CoQ10 is depleted, and the muscles cry out for more. I recommend 100 mg per day, even without cholesterol medication and up to 300 mg per day with it. The dosage required depends on the individual and on the dosage of cholesterol medication.

Adequate minerals are important, especially magnesium. Magnesium is important for more than 300 enzymatic processes in the body, most of which occur in the brain. For the heart, the best source is magnesium malate because malate helps in energy production as well.

In addition to CoQ10, magnesium, and malate, several other nutrients can impact the function of mitochondria. L-carnitine, alpha lipoic acid, many of the B-complex vitamins, manganese, and grape seed extract have helped a number of my patients. The dosage required depends on the individual.

## Environmental Strategies

Many medications that affect the heart and energy production throughout the body. If you take several medications, work with someone who is qualified to help you to find the right nutrients to replace what is lost from the medications. Almost every medication prescribed depletes vitamins and minerals. A person cannot eat enough food to replace what has been lost.

Heavy metals, like mercury, fluoride, and chlorine; insecticides and pesticides, along with electromagnetic fields and radiation, also interfere with energy production.

## Physical Strategies

Empower your epigenetic abilities and stimulate your genes with exercise. Jim is sixty-seven and stays very active year-round. In the summer, he rides his bike daily and participates in an annual bike ride across Iowa, Ragbrai. When I looked at his genetic report related to his energy production it indicated that he has 70 percent reduced function in several of the genes related to energy production, yet his energy is great. I contribute his energy to the multiple studies that indicate increased exercise increases energy production.

High-impact interval training has been shown recently to be the best way to improve physical fitness, insulin sensitivity, and mitochondrial content.[30] High intensity interval training is associated with greater impact on physical fitness, insulin sensitivity and muscle mitochondrial content in males with overweight/obesity, as opposed to continuous endurance training according to a randomized controlled trial.

## Types of Exercise

- ❖ Weight training, just one to two times per week, will increase muscle mass. If you prefer to increase muscle mass doing yoga or Pilates, those are also beneficial.
- ❖ Aerobic exercise such as walking, running, and swimming will increase strength and flexibility, but not to excess. Too much aerobic exercise is a physical stress on the body. For example it is okay to train for and run a marathon or half-marathon, but it is not good to run hours each day for years.
- ❖ High-impact interval training is the best form of exercise to improve stress handling and release weight. This type of exercise gets the heart rate up and is done in 15–20 minutes.

It is never too late to build muscle mass. In a study of seventy-plus men and women doing light resistance training, significant improvements in muscle mass were noted in the participants.[31] Slow movement resistance training using body weight improves muscle mass in the elderly.

## Eyes

The eyes are often said to be the window to the soul. We use our vision to drink in the beauty of the earth and the faces and forms of our loved ones. The vision of the face of your lover, a child's smile, a majestic mountain range, or a gorgeous sunset all stir our heart and souls. The eyes allow the light in.

We read others by looking into their eyes. We can read whether the other person is sociable, curious, happy, or contemplative. Expressive facial movements around the eyes show others our moods and emotions.

The eyes are also a window into a vision of the brain. Understanding the metabolic changes in the retina can be used not only as a biomarker for eye diseases but some prominent fatal diseases as well.

The eye is an organ of the brain, which is easily accessible and shares similar vasculature, anatomy, and physiology to the brain. Vision loss or vision changes should not be ignored or neglected. In fact, the molecular changes in the retina can be used as a biomarker of neurological diseases such as Alzheimer's, Parkinson's, and stroke, if tested appropriately.

A person who requires glasses to see at a distance, metaphorically sees the small details but could expand their vision to look at the big picture. Seeing poorly up close and requiring glasses to read or to focus on things up close necessitates looking beyond the big picture to the smaller pieces that help the world to make sense.

Most of us need reading glasses as we age. Perhaps it is a reminder that in addition to looking at the fine detail when aging, humans may have the desire to understand the big picture, and explore where they fit into this expansive universe. Aging is a time to look inward and reflect, and allow the feminine divine to share her message.

Some tips to help maintain eye health as you age.

1. Eat a balanced and healthy diet. Choose foods rich in antioxidants, like vitamins A and C; leafy, green vegetables; and fish.
2. Exercise.
3. Get a good night's sleep.
4. Wash your hands.

5. Do not smoke.
6. Wear sunglasses to protect eyes from the sun.
7. Limit use of devices that emit blue light.

My mother always told me to eat my carrots to have healthy eyes. Nutrients that support eye health are beta-carotene found in carrots and other orange and yellow vegetables that convert to vitamin A, an essential nutrient in the body.

## Mental Strategies

Have a bigger heart on a metaphorical level by helping and doing good for others, by sharing your gifts and talents, and by saying, "I love you," or showing greater outward love and affection.

## Emotional Strategies

Seek and find joy and fulfillment in personal power. Courage requires vulnerability; feeling vulnerable and taking actions anyway, along with being open to feeling big emotion.

## Relationship Strategies

Set boundaries and be willing to say no. Take responsibility for your own actions and not for the actions and emotions of others. If you don't set boundaries, you are giving yourself away. This leads to resentment, burnout, and blame. You cannot be your authentic self without boundaries.

## Creative Visualization

See your heart surrounded and infused with a pink glow filled with your love. Expand that love glow beyond your chest, beyond the room you are in, and let it radiate out to the world.

## Genetic Strategies

Divine feminine and the masculine power of the sun, with its radiant principle, means stepping into personal power and shining your divine feminine and divine masculine essence to the world in balance, and with authenticity. The power emerges by releasing the ego and stepping into the self. Radiance is being genuine and courageous. Strength and courage includes being vulnerable enough to bare the heart and soul to the world, yet also being brave enough to set boundaries.

Genetic expression is enhanced when we consistently *ask* from the heart, and *act* from the heart. It is fine to think and weigh information in the head, but actively shift those thoughts, moving that energy from the thought in the head directly to the heart space prior to making decisions or taking actions. Use the breath to shift and move the energy. Let actions and words come from the heart, carried forward with love.

Bravery is required to be vulnerable enough to feel all that life offers: the good, the bad, and the ugly. Allow the heart to feel and experience disappointment, grief, and heartache as well as joy, connection, and love.

Heartbreak will happen if we are willing to show our love. "The wound is where the light enters" as Persian poet and mystic Rumi wrote.

Allow the illumination and trust in the power of vulnerability.

## JUPITER

## EXPANSION AND SOUL GROWTH

### Associated Body Parts

> liver
> legs
> hips and hip joints

### Associated Symptoms and Diseases

> osteoarthritis of the hip
> hip dysplasia
> Perthes disease
> slipped capital femoral epiphysis
> obesity
> hepatitis
> cirrhosis
> fat accumulation in the liver (nonalcoholic fatty liver disease)
> autoimmune hepatitis
> primary biliary cholangitis
> primary sclerosing cholangitis
> genetic liver disease
> liver disease from toxins or medications
> liver cancer
> bile duct cancer
> liver adenoma
> growth of cancer in any tissue
> obesity

Obesity is the primary condition associated with the energy of Jupiter. Instead of living a more expansive, fulfilling life, people often yield to the ease and comfort of sedentary lifestyles, which include comfort foods, processed foods, and restaurant meals.

The food industry plays into our weaknesses by researching the right balance of sugar, salt, and fat to cause us to crave certain meals and flavors. These companies go to great lengths to keep us addicted. Flavor enhancers are added to many processed foods. It is well known how addictive sugar can be, so it is purposely added to many foods. Sugar is more addictive than heroin. The industrial food companies often hire overweight and obese people to test their products.[32]

I have been blessed to have the opportunity to travel to many places in the world and eat a variety of different foods. The serving sizes in restaurants in the United States are by far the largest than in any other country. The large chain restaurants in the industry cash in on the research that causes food cravings and increases obesity by making sure their offerings have the right balance of fat, salt, and sugar to keep their customers returning.

One in three adults people in the USA are considered overweight or obese, as are one in four children. These statistics are alarming due to the skyrocketing increases in diabetes and its effect on healthcare costs.[33]

I am as guilty of succumbing to comfort foods as so many others. Weight issues are a repetitive theme in my life and in my genetic heritage. I do well for periods of time, then fall into the easier way of being bigger in the world.

My extra weight is twofold. First it is partly an insulation from the pains and illness of others. I am getting better at releasing what is not mine, but I continue to struggle with caring for myself when I care for others. I get into "doctor mode," and set aside everything else. I remind myself often when I am giving others advice; "Get up more frequently when working at the computer," "Drink more water," "Exercise and stretch more." Yet at the end of a work day, I find I have not followed my own advice!

The other factor is a desire to be more expansive in my life, to experience all that life has to offer, to explore and to grow as a spiritual human being.

As I reviewed stories of people who have released a lot of weight, I am reminded of the number of people who I have been able to help most often. The people who have been successful are those who have a larger purpose, a reason to achieve the goal with a more noble cause or altruistic resolve—not one specific diet plan, though most people follow a plan for guidance.

Arlene was a food addict topping out at 305 pounds, which led to hypertension, high cholesterol, and fatty liver. She freed herself of 120 pounds when her sister was diagnosed with terminal cancer, and she needed to be there for her sister's children.

Losing both parents before the age of twenty, Martin insulated himself from his pain and loss with food. He was more than 400 pounds. He took off more than 150 pounds over a three-year period and shared that it was hard, but that it moved him to places he never thought he would be.

Maria, Jennifer, and Amy each released more than fifty pounds and became health and fitness coaches.

Chris is down twenty pounds as she moves toward her goal of becoming a motivational speaker.

Matt and Jean followed a healthy diet together prior to getting married because they wanted to look good for the wedding and more importantly, have a healthy family.

Blake wanted to let go of his excess 90 pounds, not because he wanted to lose weight but because he wanted to be healthy and play with his little brothers and participate in their lives.

Telling yourself you are going to lose weight in itself can be defeating. Losing is not expansive, it is diminishing, and words matter. The brain doesn't want to lose anything.

Decide what you want to move toward: a thinner healthier body, an active lifestyle, a dream of climbing a mountain, or becoming a marathon runner. Release the foods, the habits, and the body fat that no longer serve. Focus on the abundance of health.

A way to be more expansive and release weight is to go longer periods without eating. Being expansive about the time you go without food is a useful strategy for some. Intermittent fasting has proved to be an effective way to reduce total calories, allow the digestive tract to stay healthy, and increase longevity. Eating in a window of six or eight hours then going without food for fourteen or sixteen hours is a safe and effective strategy for most. I recommend getting the support of a health coach or physician if you want to fast for longer periods of time.[34]

Liver disease affects millions of people each year and is also related to Jupiter energy. Tim was diagnosed with hepatitis B and nonalcoholic liver cirrhosis. He was told by the medics that the condition was incurable, and he would be on medication the rest of his life. He started on the medications for about a year, but then decided he had to take a different route. The medications may slow progression of the disease, but at what cost? The liver is the primary organ that has to clear the medications, and it was already damaged.

He wrote, "During my career, I read about people miraculously healed of their diseases by the use of herbs, diet, prayer, and meditation, and although I was a believer, never had to put it in practice. Being at a crossroads of delaying the inevitable, I decided to go the holistic route. Someone I followed very closely named Edgar Cayce was instrumental in this journey and followed the advice as best as I could. I changed my diet to mostly vegetarian/vegan to decrease the strain in the liver but also provide the necessary rebuilding nutrients needed; I took herbs that encouraged liver health and elimination of toxins, exercise; I used massage to help the bodies circulation, and lots of prayer and meditation."

He did this for a year and a half before telling his medical doctor he had stopped his medication. This was after the doctor told him that his hepatitis numbers were good and the hepatitis was under control. A few months later, his physicians performed a liver scan, and there was no evidence of disease. The liver tissue had totally healed. A miracle through holistic healing!

Hip pain, also related to the Jupiter archetype, is a frequent complaint in my chiropractic practice. A common location for degenerative changes, hip replacements are frequent, and hip fractures are common. After a hip fracture, the one-year mortality rate in the elderly ranges from 14 to 58 percent.[35] In usual care, the reported one-year mortality after sustaining a hip fracture has been estimated to be 14 to 58 percent. The relative risk of mortality in the elderly patient population increases 4 percent per year. The first year after a hip fracture is a critical time. Since hip fracture represents forward momentum it can signal the beginning of the end of life. The issues are important.

In a conversation with Marcia after her chiropractic treatment, I learned she has chronic low back aches and pain along with achy, stiff hips. She lives alone with her two toy poodles and just celebrated sixty-eight years. She has one daughter and a grandson she adores. Her daughter was recently fired from her job because she was going to have to have back surgery for a herniated disc, causing intense pain in her back and radiating to her foot. She had been waiting for this back surgery and was fired because she needed two weeks off.

Marcia, who has very little money of her own, has been stretching her budget to help her daughter make house payments. She doesn't want her to lose her house during this time. She had been unemployed for several weeks.

This limited income affected both women. Marcia's daughter is in constant pain and she, like most mothers, hates to see her suffer; she longs to alleviate her daughter's pain.

We got to talking about what lower back pain has to do feelings of being supported, and hip pain and hip motion relate to forward momentum. I suggested that perhaps part of her personal pain relays the message that Marcia is taking on some of her daughter's pain and problems. Marcia wanted to help her in a larger way but was unable to do so, not unlike a lot of mothers, including me. I always want to nurture my babies and relieve their pain, no matter their age. It doesn't matter whether it is possible or not, the desire remains and the desire affects us.

I have known Marcia a long time and know that she is Catholic and has a great faith and religious practice. I reminded her that she is not alone. A higher power is there to help carry some of this burden. Could she hand over more of her pain and the resolution of the problems to the higher power she believes in? Could she grow her faith with trust that everything will work out for the best?

A person doesn't need to have a great religious faith to hand over their troubles to a higher power. Any spiritual belief of an organizing force in the universe will do. A belief in cosmic consciousness: To whom it may concern.

Share with others the burden of troubles to create a community of those who can help, support, and hold space for important feelings. Allow others to hold your intentions and/or pray on your behalf. This is not a time to go it alone. Community and connection is an important aspect of embracing the divine feminine.

Return troubles and burdens to Mother Earth, the source of all the elements that make our bodies. The earth is solid and firm and has the capacity to hold all the healing waters and all humanity. This is a way of balancing the masculine fire of Jupiter with the feminine nurturing and healing energy of the earth. People study crystals and the healing power of different kinds of stones for different purposes.

Try this strategy: Simply take a stone, a solid chunk of earth, and blow troubles and worries into it. The stone has the capacity to carry the burden, it has no emotional attachment, and can lighten the weight of the emotion or pain that is carried. One doesn't have to be alone or carry troubles alone.

People known as empaths easily take on the pain and burdens of others but often with a physical or emotional cost. It is a wonderful gift to feel so deeply, yet empaths must continually use tools to keep emotions flowing *through* rather than *carry* the pain and emotions of others. Stuck emotions can feel like a heaviness, a weight, strings tugging at the heart, or an energetic buzzing feeling. Some feel the actual physical pain of others.

Breathe into your heart space and feel grateful for the ability to have this type of expansive love, however I know that the pain and emotions of others require movement and flow. When I am feeling the energy of others, even after they have left me and moved on, I use water to wash that heavy energy away. Washing my hands with the intention of washing away their energy allows me to feel lighter.

Jupiter energy also has to do with the growth of cancer. Cancer growth is growth and expansion, but at the wrong level. The origin or causes of cancer is usually related to the energy of other archetypes or in exposure to environmental chemicals, yet its growth is in Jupiter. Those who heal or have remission from cancer have done much more than radiation, chemo, or surgery. They have increased their research to look for alternative ways to heal and expanded their horizons to new ways of healing. They often have healed from broken relationships and grown their faith in higher powers. Their wisdom is magnified and expanded in ways that were incomprehensible to those who have not experienced cancer.

Unfortunately, those who have cancer treatments often grow in understanding of suffering and pain. Cancer patients also grow their understanding of fear, anxiety, and the concept of fighting. Fighting seems to be the terminology associated with the medical approach to cancer treatment. Cancer is a battle to be fought and won. You are forever identified as a cancer patient in the middle of a battle.

Cancer is part of the body and has a message. Yes, one must aggressively search out the conflicts that allowed the onset and assertively take the dramatic actions required to change the environment and the expression in the body—not a situation to be taken lightly. In addition to working with medical professionals that you trust, ask the cancer, "In what ways do I need to expand and grow as a spiritual vessel to expand my meaning and purpose in this life or to grow as an individual?"

If you are unsure of this answer, seek spiritual guidance or psychological help to uncover what is held within.

Regrettably, cancer is one of the leading causes of death, and I have lost many family members, patients, and friends to various forms of cancer. Some never have the opportunity to ask any questions or have any time to heal. I encourage all my patients who have had or recovered from cancer to continue on the path of self-growth and understanding. Each one of my patients with a cancer diagnosis, when questioned, have said they learned many valuable lessons from their cancer.

Prevention occurs when we address all the conflicts we are able to observe and illuminate aspects that are held within us as we continue to grow as the spiritual beings that we are.

## Nutritional Strategies

Since we are talking about expansion, let's explore the expanded use of vegetables. I am overwhelmed by the number of people who tell me they don't like vegetables.

"Get over it!" said one of my nutrition instructors. I agree. Our bodies like the color, the nutrients, and the fiber that vegetables offer us.

A lot of people don't like vegetables because they haven't had them prepared well. If the only experience is like mine, Mom opening a can of peas and expected me to like them. No wonder. My mother frequently burned vegetables she poured out of the can and still served them to the family. Talk about disgusting! Surprising that I ever learned to enjoy vegetables.

Experiment with different methods of preparation; use spice blends, and play with seasonings you like on other foods. Stir fry, roast, or grill them. Chop veggies into tiny pieces, or puree them and add to sauces and soups. Explore recipes. The possibilities are endless. Be expansive when it comes to veggies.

If overweight, choose veggies that are lower in glycemic index. The glycemic index is how quickly a food breaks down to sugar in the bloodstream. This is why people who are releasing weight limit the potatoes and corn, vegetables high in glycemic index. One can eat lots of low glycemic veggies, even on a reduced carbohydrate diet.

## Environmental Strategies

Use caution in restaurants. Limit restaurant meals with huge serving sizes and added chemicals for food freshness. Use caution, as buffet tables often use added chemicals to keep the food appearing fresh for hours. If the serving size is huge, plan to take some home to eat later.

## Physical Strategies

Auriculotherapy and reflexology are methods to use the small to activate the large. Points on the ear and on the hands and feet relate to all parts of the body.

## Emotional Strategies

Practice big emotions in no-risk situations. Use these strategies to build personal confidence.

- Practice crying and grief by watching a sad movie.
- Practice courage by watching a movie about someone overcoming a major obstacle.

## Relationship Strategies

Speak slowly, use minimal words. The brain cannot hear more than about twenty words at a time. This gives others a chance to truly hear you and what you have to say. This is the advice of author and neuroscientist, Mark Waldman.

## Mental Strategies

In keeping with the advice of Mark Waldman, write out a CRAP list, a listing of all the **C**onflicts, **R**esistance, **A**nxieties, and **P**rocrastinations or problems held within. Be sure to include at least twenty doubts, worries, weaknesses, or limiting beliefs, real or imaginary.

Relax deeply as you gaze at the list. Yawn and stretch while continuing to gaze at the list. Ask your intuition what else should be added to the list, what weaknesses do you believe others would say you have? Add those things to the list.

Keep gazing at the list while continuing to deeply relax. Yawn and stretch several times. If comfortable, gently stroke your hands and arms, which stimulates areas of the brain related to self-confidence and calms emotions. Notice the negative emotions related to all the CRAP has reduced in intensity.

Don't throw the CRAP away! Put it up on the wall where it can be seen frequently. On the wall, the CRAP is safely stored, and you can add to it if necessary.

Over time, fewer negative thoughts will be noticed. Discarding the list allows the unconscious mind to reflect and ruminate and pick up all that negative thought once again.

Mark Waldman suggests, "Remember: Old memories are always 'there' in your brain, but you don't have to listen to them or believe they are true. You can even talk to them and tell them to 'shut up.' They usually will. Then focus on your three deepest values for that day, and the new belief you want to embed into your memory."

## Creative Visualization

See yourself strolling along a path when you see someone walking toward you. They come closer and you realize it is you, but a slightly older you, three years from now, who is radiant and healthy. Ask your future self what it took to achieve this future and what advice they want to give you. Take your time and experience all that you can. Thank them for sharing and for being willing to make this transformation.

## Genetic Strategies

Expanding our soul and consciousness requires us to tap into personal beliefs. To examine and illuminate the areas where expansion is good and desirable.

Life is often lived with blinders, going through the motions, meeting one crisis after another, not examining anything. The US is a nation of overconsumption with more foods that lead to obesity, more money for more material possessions, larger homes, and bigger cars. Our society drives a desire for more and more money and more stuff; yet is that the true desire? Perhaps the desire for stuff hides a desire to be more fulfilled, more satisfied, safer, or more accepted.

Hidden are the feelings of inadequacy related to doing enough, being enough, or having enough. These thought patterns were set into our genes from the struggles of our ancestors. Have awareness and catch when your thoughts go to autopilot. Our ancestors likely had to work from daybreak to sunset and still often went hungry or lacked material possessions. My parents were raised during the Depression when millions of people lacked food and/or the ability to produce income. This instilled in them a poverty mentality. My father often told the story of his mother crying on the side of the road because she found a dime, and that meant she could feed the children that day. My mother saved everything in case she might need it someday.

Some of the actions that will expand the part of you that is a divine spiritual being are growing wisdom, faith, and deep trust, expanding insight, enthusiasm, and optimism—also growing a sense of justice, and building bridges of tolerance and connection.

We can epigenetically strengthen and trust the thoughts that we really are enough, do enough, and have enough.

## CHAPTER SIX
# WATER ARCHETYPES

## Water

Water is known as the universal solvent. It dissolves more substances than any other liquid. It can dissolve salt, sugar, acids, alkalis, and some minerals, gasses, and organic materials. This ability to dissolve has helped the ocean dissolve the $CO_2$ produced from the burning of fossil fuels and process it with sea vegetation. This keeps the atmosphere healthy. Traveling through the world in streams and rivers, water carries minerals, chemicals, and nutrients with it. The abundant water on this planet has supported life by keeping the temperatures in a narrow, yet comfortable, range because it takes a long time to shift water temperatures. Planets without water, like Mercury, experience huge shifts in temperatures, depending on what side faces the sun. We don't experience those extremes. Hopefully we can keep it that way as we are seeing changes with global warming. Now with global warming the ocean temperatures are rising. As of last month, the North Atlantic was 2 degrees Fahrenheit above its historical average.

Water supports and cleans air, drowns out fires, and dissolves earth. Observe the deep canyons created by rivers and streams. Yet we need the earth to be a container for the water. Water always requires a container.

The human body is approximately 60 percent water and, depending on the tissue, has even a higher percentage. Water is essential to life. A person can go about three weeks without food but only three to four days without water.

Just as in rivers and streams, water in the body carries chemicals, minerals, and nutrients to all parts of the body.

"The solution to pollution is dilution," says my mentor, Dr. Bob Rakowski, so having adequate water helps to keep the human tissues and rivers and streams clearing waste and environmental chemicals.

Water is associated with emotions. Words that express the element of water are intuitive, reflective, transcendent, emotional, sensitive, mysterious, or refreshing.

Imbalanced water can result in moodiness, victimhood, revenge, dependence, addiction, destruction, self-destruction, hypersensitivity, instability, drowning, and disassociation. The person can be easily hurt or offended and may be inclined to blame others.

# MOON

# NURTURING AND REFLECTING

## Associated Body Parts

- breasts
- mouth
- stomach
- vagina
- uterus
- ovaries

## Associated Symptoms and Diseases

- breast pain, the most-commonly associated with swelling breast tissue during the menstrual cycle
- gynecomastia
- cysts
- fibroadenomas
- fat necrosis
- sclerosing adenosis
- generalized breast lumpiness
- breast tenderness
- breast cancer
- dysmenorrhea
- endometriosis
- uterine fibroids
- gynecologic cancer
- HIV/AIDS
- interstitial cystitis
- polycystic ovary syndrome (PCOS)
- sexually transmitted diseases (STDs)
- pelvic inflammatory disease (PID)
- prolapsed uterus
- vaginitis
- vaginal infection from yeast, bacteria, or parasite

## Digestion

GERD
gastritis
peptic ulcer
gastroenteritis
hiatal hernia
gastroparesis
stomach cancer

The full moon, bright in the sky, is reflecting and sparkling on the still, dark lake. The light is absorbed into the depths of the water, magical and powerful, pulling my heartstrings and stirring my soul. The moon, so powerful, creates tides, cycles, and rhythms. Throughout history, moon energy has been considered female, and I sense that rhythm as I watch the moon rise over the water. The water is soaking up and absorbing the light and the power of the moon, just as I am, absorbing the energy of the moon and reflecting on its power as I rock back and forth on the porch swing.

Water is feminine energy. Feminine energy is internal, what we take in: inside, into the dark, into the part of us that reflects, listens, absorbs, examines, and explores, going directly into the dark, into the shadow.

People, including myself, have difficulty looking within and looking at the shadow. We would rather watch a horror movie about shadowy creatures than ever examine what shadows lurk within. Yet there is a benefit to looking within.

Innumerable beautiful things within the body occur in darkness. *Every thought that you think, every breath that you take, every bit of food that you digest, and every beat of your heart occurs in the darkness.*

The darkness, the shadow, is a beautiful place. Sometimes we tuck some unexamined emotions into the deep recesses only to have them emerge later, but it is nothing to fear. If we change our perception and look at our shadow as the inside of the body, the interior aspect of our human experience, it becomes awesome.

The inside of the body talks to us all the time, as noted in previous chapters. But the moon, what is its language? As I watch the moon on the water, I think of Betty.

Betty glances at the clock, "Oh s***; I'm running late again."

It's 6:00 a.m. and she really should have been out of bed a half-hour ago. She calls up the stairs to her two beautiful daughters, Emily, fourteen, and Brooke, sixteen, that they need to be at volleyball practice in less than forty-five minutes, and they better get a move on.

Thank goodness they put in the extra bath last year, or she would never be able to get ready in time. She jumps in the shower, throws on her clothes and makeup. She has to be dressed for the office before she drops off the girls, or she will never be to work in time.

With a board meeting today, she must have all the board packets done and on the table before the meeting. She had them almost done before she left last night, but there was a volleyball game that she had to get to that was an hour away.

She can't miss a ball game, can she?

Her job, the executive assistant for a professional organization, usually allows a little flexibility with her hours, but today is that meeting, and Brooke has to be to dance practice by 3:30. Both girls have to be back to school by 5:30 tonight for the volleyball game. No time for breakfast for herself, Betty yells to the girls that it is time to go, hands them each a granola bar, grabs her coffee, and dashes to the car.

Betty reported to me on her nutrition visit that she has chronic indigestion and takes a prescription antacid each day. She has heavy, painful menstrual cycles and frequent bladder infections that require antibiotics. She is fifty pounds overweight and has back pain and recurrent migraine headaches.

The astrological archetype of the moon is associated with pregnancy and the womb, fertility, motherhood, and motherly love. Creating cozy comfortable places, nurturing the family, and feeding and nurturing the children are also moon tasks. In addition to caring for others, the task of the moon is to allow space to nurture and to care for oneself, the psyche, and the inner child.

Betty is at a difficult time in life when it is so difficult to find any balance or rhythm. She is allowing life to set her rhythm rather than setting her own, and she feels like a victim. She is great at nurturing her children, but has totally neglected her need to nurture herself.

The rhythm of life is an important theme of the moon, just as it is with the sun. We need rhythm in our lives, and the female menstrual cycle is the classic example of such rhythm. In a world without artificial light, women's menstrual cycles would naturally be in sync with the cycle of the moon and in conjunction with each other.

Diseases associated with the moon include diseases in the cave-like areas of the body such as the stomach, the mouth, and the bladder. Most prominent are the diseases of the soft, round, organs of fertility and nurturing; the breasts, uterus, and ovaries.

Betty's girls have club volleyball this weekend in Omaha, so this time will cost more, with the hotel room and the restaurant. Club volleyball is twice a month, but sometimes they are close enough to drive home after the games. She is not looking forward to the eight hours on Saturday and the four hours on Sunday, sitting on bleachers.

When is she going to get the laundry done? It is piling up.

Betty is so tired. There are ball games at least three days this week due to volleyball season. It won't stop, because volleyball is followed by basketball season and softball season. Tonight she will get home at 9:30 or 10:00 p.m. Her husband Tim will meet her at the games, and they will grab supper at the snack bar. Oh boy, another meal of walking tacos or hotdogs and chips. She will let the Diet Pepsi keep her going.

It's 10:00 p.m. when she gets home, and Betty sends the kids off to homework and bed. When she finally sits, she realizes she is starving. She gets up, walks to the kitchen, stares into the fridge, wondering what to eat. She gobbles some cheese and crackers and a few glasses of wine to wash it down. She deserves it, doesn't she? It has been such a long, tough day.

Betty knows she sacrifices for the kids, but it is so damn hard. No way around it. Emily will need a new pair of shoes next week; another hundred bucks, and then there are the uniforms and the next hotel bill. In a few years, the kids will be grown, then maybe she will have more time and more money. She knows she needs to eat better and to get more exercise, but how can she? There are no more hours in her day.

Betty's body is screaming at her, calling out for nurturance and attention. Her shadow, her psyche, the inside of her body is asking for self-love, play, kindness, and care. She is unable and unwilling to look within, to reflect on what her body is telling her.

I understand Betty so well because I have been there too, feeling like a victim to circumstances, and giving more that I had to give. Her story is such a similar pattern to scores of my female patients, the mothers, the teachers, and counselors who have come to see me over the years.

Betty drifts off while watching some late-night reruns. She startles herself awake and finds herself alone, cold, asleep in her chair with the drone of the TV in the background. Tim went to bed hours ago. His day starts at 4:00 a.m. She shuts it all down and heads off to bed, feeling agitated and irritable. It is 2:00 a.m.

Current epidemics of breast cancer and infertility hint at our society's lack of respect for the moon and its feminine qualities. Western medicine practices are quick to use interventions that control and manage menstrual cycles and medicate upset stomachs. Surgeons cut off or cut out the organs of fertility as opposed to finding alternative solutions.

Western patriarchal society expects women to give of themselves at the expense of good health. Attention and nurturing is given to jobs, children, families, homes, and mortgages, long before attention and nurturing is given to the self.

Betty has the opportunity to transform and become whole and connected to herself and her needs, if she chooses to take action to do so. Unfortunately, I couldn't supplement her horrible diet or change things for Betty. She was the one who needed to ask for help and take the actions to change. I attempted to work with her, but she could see no way that she could eat better, move more, or to carve out time for self-care. It was easier to take the prescribed medications.

I hope that Betty will see her way to finding ways to feed her soul and her body in meaningful ways, once her children are grown, and she has more time for herself. To take as much as she gives. To create a balance of the masculine, giving out energy, and the feminine, receiving energy. To release her need to feel the victim. Her body will continue to talk, whether she is or isn't ready to listen.

A person with balanced moon energy feels connected, empathetic, sees their potential, and nourishes their inner child. This is water energy, like the moon reflecting on water, and the tides moving the water. Men and women alike need to reflect, absorb, examine, explore, and to create their own rhythm . Each person can nurture, whether it is a child, a relationship, an animal, or a creative endeavor. It benefits each of us to nurture our inner child; the original, true nature, childlike aspects of the individual.

People with moon imbalance often feel victim to life, project their problems on others, are often offended, feel moody, have trouble making decisions, and can be very dependent.

Mary, age fifty-two, has short, brown hair and a cheerful smile. She was due for a routine mammogram, and cancer was discovered in her right breast. She runs her own marketing business, and this cancer was discovered just after she settled a lawsuit against her that had been going on for the previous three years.

The lawsuit was an ugly situation that had been foremost in her mind for that whole time. She experienced a level of stress and anxiety she was unable to control during those years. Her body accustomed itself to be on chronic alert, habitually pumping out the chemicals of stress while she attempted to keep her business going and manage the lawsuit. She often found herself feeling the victim of her circumstance.

It's easy to visualize the environment that created breast cancer in Mary. She was able to just have a lumpectomy, so the surgery and healing time was minimal. Mary changed her diet and switched to eating only organic foods. She added healthy nutrients, along with allowing herself time to nurture her female aspects. She incorporated time for reflection, self-care, self-nurturing.

As a business owner, mother, and spouse, she looked at the balance between receiving and giving. The time of introspection, as she was healing from her breast surgery, was something that has been sorely lacking in the previous years. It was vital for her healing process.

A year later, she is feeling great and knows she has healed what created the problem in the first place.

Sometimes it is difficult to understand why we feel like victims and why we have trouble with others. We give over our power to others. Mona slumped into the chair in front of me, "I hate that woman!"

"What woman?" I asked.

Mona went into a tirade about the woman at her work who always bullied and degraded her. "This woman is ruining a perfectly good job for me."

She told me that the boss was great and fair, but this woman was making her job miserable.

We discussed the possibility of processing these feelings in a different way. Did she really want to give this bully coworker so much power over her life? No one should be able to make your life miserable or make you feel like a victim.

Our own reactions to situations make our lives miserable, not the situations themselves.

Byron Katie wrote, "Who would you be, how would you react, without that thought?" Do we want to remain miserable, or do we want to shift the thought?

Byron Katie explores forgiveness in her four questions when faced with a dilemma or frustration with a specific issue:[36]

Ask yourself:

> *Is it true?*
> *Can I absolutely know that it is true?*
> *How do I react when I believe that thought?*
> *Who would I be without that thought?*

If one can release from the thoughts, the thoughts that make us unhappy, a shift can occur in perception.

I asked Mona if she ever bullied or berated someone. She thought about it for a while and was able to come up with a couple of situations where her words were harsh and unkind. We discussed the concepts of shadow and projection. Shadow is what we are unable to perceive within ourselves. Perhaps she was seeing in others the things about herself that she really didn't like. That is projection. She admitted that she was rather stubborn and severe at times, and she could bully and berate herself, especially when she was fearful.

My suggestion was to begin to perceive this coworker in a different light. Perhaps her attack on Mona was not really directed at Mona. Perhaps her coworker was attacking herself. Perhaps her outburst was a self-criticism or self-assault. She likely was unhappy with herself, didn't like aspects of herself, and needed to vent.

Perhaps the projection went both ways. Mona can continue to react to this woman and allow her the power to influence her job and work environment or she can send love and forgiveness to the woman and realize that her attacks are not personal.

Stomach issues related to this archetype are often due to stress. The body will shunt energy away from the digestive tract to "run away from the tiger," and in response the body doesn't make enough enzymes to break down foods.

If we listen to the media, the doctors and the drug companies, we hear that people have too much acid, which is rarely correct. It takes a significant amount of acid (a very acid pH of 2 or 3) to get food broken down in the stomach and allow the food to leave the stomach.

If we are stressed or depleted, the stomach struggles to lower its pH to the appropriate level and sits there in the stomach at a pH of 3.5 to 4.5, which is still acid, enough to upset the stomach, but not enough to support digestion. It leaves but just trickles out. Unfortunately, if the food is not at the right pH, it won't stimulate the liver and gallbladder to release bile to break down fats, or the pancreas and small intestine to release enzymes to break down proteins and the rest of the carbohydrates. Ineffective, insufficient stomach acid affects the absorption of many nutrients from foods or supplements.

A few people have too much stomach acid, but they are rare. It takes a lot of body energy to change food from a pH of 6 or 7 all the way to a pH of 2 to 3. Most people I observe do not complain of having too much energy.

The medical approach is to give the patient antacids or proton-pump inhibitors, which further lower the digestive ability of the stomach. It takes away the burning but only covers the problem. They are designed to be taken for a short period of time, yet I have seen people on these medications for twenty or more years. The body eventually can no longer make stomach acid.

Stomach acid is required for breaking down calcium. Interesting that many people who take antacids for many years develop osteopenia and osteoporosis.

## Nutritional Strategies

Supplements can boost stomach acid while you are learning strategies to deal with stress. Betaine HCL, 300–750 mg, taken at the beginning of the meal will boost stomach acid and stimulate digestion. Often digestive formulations combine betaine HCL with pepsin the chief digestive enzyme in the stomach, which breaks down proteins into polypeptides.

Betaine HCL is only to be taken with food, *never* on an empty stomach. If it causes burning, it is totally neutralized with some baking soda in water. This means your stomach lining needs some healing and repair before you can use betaine HCL.

A person shouldn't have to take enzymes forever. Once a person starts to digest better, they often absorb the nutrients that make enzymes in the first place and the Betaine HCL is no longer needed.

## Foods and nutrients that will speed healing and repair of the digestive tract:

L-glutamine, an amino acid that helps with repair of the gut lining
seafood, such as fish, mussels, shrimps, and crabs
grass-fed meat
red cabbage
milk
eggs
yogurt
ricotta cheese
nuts

Taking L-glutamine as a supplement may be necessary to heal the digestive tract for some with serious conditions.

Aloe vera and okra can both help heal and protect the lining of the digestive tract and are safe and effective with rare side effects.

Deglycyrrhizinated licorice, licorice (glycyrrhiza glabra) is a soothing anti-inflammatory herb. The active part of the plant is the root and has a long history of medicinal use, especially in Asia. In DGL, glycyrrhizin has been removed as it can cause elevations in blood pressure. DGL is used for heartburn (acid reflux) and stomach inflammation. It relieves symptoms and repairs the lining of the digestive tract. Some find taking one 400 mg chewable tablet twenty minutes prior to meals or before bedtime is effective. DGL is safe in the above doses with no significant side effects.

If you have a family history or history of breast cancer, it is a good idea to eat a half-cup serving each day of anything in the brassica group of veggies to help toxic estrogens from plastics and pesticides to be eliminated from the body through healthy pathways. These foods are broccoli, Brussels sprouts, cabbage, cauliflower, kohlrabi, kale, or other variations of that family of foods.[37] Brassica vegetable consumption shifts estrogen metabolism in healthy postmenopausal women. The beneficial effects of brassica vegetables on human health.

Adequate B-complex vitamins especially if you are taking birth control or hormone replacement. These medications deplete B vitamins faster than you can get them in. Deficiencies in folate, just one of the many B vitamins depleted by birth control, is associated with increased risk of cancer, diabetes, stroke, heart disease, depression, and neural tube defects in infants.[38]

Some women require evening primrose or borage oils, the anti-inflammatory omega-6 essential fatty acids, to stimulate healthy prostaglandin production.

## Creative Visualization

If possible, reflect on the ways you were nurtured and on the ways you felt as if there was something lacking. If there are still feelings of lack or loss, is it possible to nurture that inner child now in healthy and fulfilling ways?

Close your eyes and visualize yourself as a young child sitting with the adult you. Have a conversation with your inner child, telling them that you are sorry they didn't get what they wanted or needed. Soothe the inner child and tell this child that you, now an adult, will care for it and provide for its needs now.

## Gratitude Practice

This can be anything from saying prayers of gratitude at night to writing down three things or more that you are grateful for each day.

"Gratitude turns what we have into enough, and more. It turns denial into acceptance, chaos into order, confusion into clarity... it makes sense of our past, brings peace for today, and creates a vision for tomorrow."

—Melody Beattie

## Emotional Strategies

Practice self-care and self-therapies. Develop a full toolbox of activities that are nourishing, reflective, creative, or peaceful. Try out different options until you find what fulfills you. Make it a priority and carve out the time. Be the example for the family. Examples are more powerful than empty words.

## Relationship Strategy

Decide the most important issues. Does it really matter if the laundry is folded a specific way, if the dishwasher is loaded a specific way, or if the toothpaste is squeezed from the bottom?

If it really matters to your inherited perfectionist tendencies, then fold the clothes, load the dishwasher, and buy a second tube of toothpaste. However, it is unfair and perhaps unreasonable to feel like a victim when doing the chores yourself. That someone doesn't do things the way you want them to doesn't mean they don't love you; they may simply be oblivious.

## Mental Strategy

Find or create a healthy rhythm for life to have a fuller expression of life. The heart rhythm and the female menstrual cycles are examples of organ systems that require healthy rhythm. Problems in these areas indicate life is out of rhythm and balance. Set your own rhythm, dance to your own drummer, not one set by others or by a sense of obligation.

## Environmental Strategy

Avoid xenoestrogens. Limit exposure to plastics and pesticides associated with xenoestrogens, toxic estrogens that imbalance hormones in the body.

## Physical Strategy

Meditation and nature walks would be a great way to tune in to what it is that you want and need. Creative projects and activities are an excellent way to maintain good health.

## Genetic Strategy

Epigenetically, besides eating the broccoli and cauliflower as mentioned, dig in and examine conscious agreements vs unconscious agreements, e.g., some of your childhood core beliefs may cause you to accept certain genetic weaknesses or have attitudes that would lead to diabetes, heart disease, or cancer; and then choose lifestyles that actually drives disease. "My dad died of a heart attack at forty-five so I probably will too, so it doesn't matter if I drink and smoke." This also applies to attitudes toward others, the unconscious agreements that create racism and prejudice.

## PLUTO

## METAMORPHOSIS

### Associated Body Parts

colon

### Associated Symptoms and Diseases

autoimmune diseases
fibromyalgia,
chronic Lyme disease
multiple sclerosis
cancer
constipation
yeast infection/overgrowth

Jan visited the office, complaining of all-over body pain. Her neck felt like tight ropes, the tightness spreading to each shoulder. The knots in her shoulder blades felt like rocks, and she yelped in pain as I gently touched them. The lower back and buttocks were just as rigid, taut, and tender. She complained of headache, lethargy, chronic constipation, and weakness. Sleep is frequently disturbed as she wakes up so many times in the night, because staying still in one place triggers pain. She wakes up as exhausted as when she went to bed. She is now taking blood pressure medication, and recently the medical doctor added an antacid.

She has come for a Band-Aid, a temporary relief from a little of her pain.

I see her as a woman stuck, allowing the ravages and desolate feelings of her life stay in control. She is living her life as a martyr.

Jan says she loves her husband, but they don't talk, and they really don't enjoy doing things together or being together. They have been married for thirty-five years, but she says they have nothing in common but the kids. No intimacy or connection.

Jan helps to run the family business and feels as if no one ever takes her feelings or needs into consideration. She allows her husband and other family members to use up her time and energy. She runs the errands, keeps up the house, and does all the cooking and cleaning. She does all the buying and ordering for the busy business. She can't be gone without telling everyone where she is going. She doesn't feel as if she can say no.

The only boundary she sets on her time is that she waits until late morning to go to the store; yet when home in the mornings she is either babysitting for grandchildren or working on the business books, or both. She is resigned to staying in this relationship, one that brings her no joy or fulfillment. She is resigned to being pushed around by her family members, using up her life for their purposes.

She accepts resignation and resentfulness as her life path. She won't even see the possibility of her life being any other way. She is in chronic pain and takes four different medications. Her life situation is stagnant with bitterness, tinged with despair.

Jan's life reminds me of a scene in the movie, *The African Queen*, starring Humphrey Bogart and Katherine Hepburn.

Katherine Hepburn plays the lonely sister of an African missionary at the beginning of World War I. This missionary and his sister live in a remote African village at the beginning of the film. Humphrey Bogart plays a steam river boat captain, running supplies up and down the river. When soldiers appear in the village and kill her brother, prim and proper Katherine is forced to go with the unsophisticated boat captain on an adventure in his boat, the African Queen, down the river. It is a great story and one of my favorite movies, a must-see for any movie buff.

The scene I am referring to is when the boat is stuck in dark, stagnant water, completely surrounded by tall reeds, no current and no channel. The two of them had been plowing deeper into the stagnant water for about two days. They have to get out of the boat and pull the boat along, even though the swampy waters are filled with leeches, and the damp humid air is filled with insects. In this scene they gave up; the boat could be pulled no farther. They resigned themselves to dying, stuck in the swamp, in the cocoon of the African Queen, never again seeing the light of day.

They fall asleep, and the scene shifts to a major storm occurring up river. Lightning, thunder, and lots of rain. We see the water levels rising all the way down the river, even though it didn't rain anywhere near where the African Queen was. The water levels rise and the Queen floats free, back into a channel, entering the lake of their destination. They are saved.

It took a major storm and shifting, flowing water to get them out of their dilemma. A metamorphosis was required to change the energy of stuck Pluto energy.

Jan's situation is not going to improve with half-hearted efforts. Her health and her life will not change if she stays stuck in the swamp of bitterness and resentment that is her life.

Pluto of Scorpio and the patterns associated can feel like a murky swamp filled with stinging insects and biting spiders. In the murky shadows are snakes and alligators, eels and leeches. Occasionally you come across a pool of cannibal fish.

Pluto is where we see the greatest contrast, the dark quagmire of treachery, treason, destruction, and especially self-destruction.

> "Most people are afraid of suffering. But suffering is a kind of mud to help the lotus flower of happiness grow. There can be no lotus flower without the mud."
> ~Thich Nhat Hanhasda

The opposite, the other end of the spectrum, contains metamorphosis, self-discipline, miracle transformations, and the phoenix rising out of the ashes. The feelings associated with Pluto have the greatest polarization and opposition, meaning the depth of shadow and the brightest illumination.

Hurting others for the sake of pleasure is at one end of the spectrum, and the glorious lotus growing out of the darkness of the swamp as the self-actualized person is at the other end of the spectrum. A self-actualized person is defined as one who has reached full potential and is authentic, self-accepting, realistic, autonomous, secure, and unashamed.

No one is without shadow and the darkness within. Everyone has moments when they feel as if the world is against them, misunderstood, and as if they will never escape the difficulties of life.

Female aggression, as mentioned in the chapter on the divine feminine, is linked to Pluto energy. Wherever the body is attacking itself it is Pluto energy. autoimmune diseases, fibromyalgia, Lyme disease, and multiple sclerosis are examples. Healing from these conditions requires radical lifestyle change.

Cancer also necessitates dramatic change to heal. Cancer is the environment of Pluto, the dark swamp of bitterness, resentment, and self-destruction, that initiates the onset of many cancers. Recovery from cancer or autoimmune disease won't work with half-hearted effort. Most often sweeping lifestyle changes, emotional shifts, and radical treatments are necessary.

Terry Wahls, in her book about healing from multiple sclerosis, *The Wahls Protocol*, wrote about a dramatic lifestyle change especially in the form of diet and supplements. The most dramatic results seen in people are those who are ready to do whatever it takes to be healed. One must be ready to address all aspects, all the conflicts. Half-hearted, wishy-washy efforts just are not up to the task of transformative change.

Sabotage, back-stabbing, treachery, horrible destruction, and self-destruction are found in the dark end of this archetype. Self-sabotage can be as simple as the food you choose to eat. Eating for pleasure even when you know the choice is horrible for you. It can also mean staying in relationships or jobs where there has been physiological or psychological damage. Situations where abuse occurs, or where you don't feel heard or cared for.

Health challenges can begin when a person's focus is on pleasure for the sake of pleasure, gluttony, and seeking things or relationships that are superficial. Participating in sex for the sake of sex, not for a meaningful connection or being in an unequal relationship where one partner wants casual sex, and one wants a deeper bond. There are so many types of toxic relationships; partners who injure each other physically or emotionally or hurt each other with lying and cheating. These situations can often go wrong, creating heartache and internal self-destruction.

One in six American women is raped during their lifetime.[39] Rape is an injury that can cause a lifetime disruption of stress mechanisms in the body, leading to greater chance of illness or psychological damage.

We find many examples of Pluto energy in our popular culture. Movies and television shows often have characters that are sick, twisted people who enjoy inflicting pain on others: blackmail, back-stabbing, physical harm, and murder. Maybe okay in a novel or a movie, but devastating in real life.

Work in environments where the exchange is not even illustrates Pluto energy. Inequities between management and the worker, child labor, and the sex worker who is often dependent on drugs are further examples.

The movie, *Pretty Woman*, is a classic example of a metamorphosis for both primary characters. The lead characters, played by Richard Gere and Julia Roberts, were each selling themselves for money. She was selling her body, and he was selling his integrity for the pursuit of money. The changes for both of them occurred when they "saved each other" with the realization of how similar their lives were. Together they could move to a life of greater integrity and self-respect.

Lori arrived at my office on a late winter day, cold, bleak, and gray. Lori's eyes and demeanor echoed that bleakness, mirroring the day. Her skin was ashen, and she had dark circles under her eyes that told me it had been weeks since she had a good night's sleep. We sat and reviewed her case history.

Lori had seen multiple doctors and had every test imaginable. She had blood tests, stool tests, hormone tests, nutrition tests, and more. She had been prescribed sleeping pills, depression and anxiety medications, and numerous natural products, but she still felt exhausted and stressed. Her gut was frequently bloated, and she had chronic constipation. She sat quietly yet it was obvious she was uncomfortable and fidgety.

Her medical doctors played with diagnosis of fibromyalgia, Lyme disease, and chronic fatigue syndrome. They had no clue. There was no definitive diagnosis. She couldn't remember the last day she felt good. She wasn't making any progress, and she feared for her future.

Lori, age forty-eight, worked as a receptionist at a large corporation. She had missed so many days in the past year that she feared she would lose her job. Fortunately, she had a job with excellent benefits and a fair number of sick days, but the days were running out, and her boss had increased the complaints about the missed days.

On her thirty-minute commute to work, Lori often had to pull over to the side of the road to rest for a few minutes before continuing the drive home at the end of the work day. Her husband Nick drove her to and from work many days even though his job took him in the opposite direction. Sometimes they just met halfway, and he took her back to the car in the morning.

Other than work, Lori stays home most of the time because adding extra activities exhausts her. She has one daughter who lives in Texas, but she has three stepsons and four grandchildren. She wants to go to ballgames and concerts but it exhausts her for a week if she does too much.

Weekends mean staying at home and resting a lot. Her energy must be preserved and protected. She is frustrated that she cannot go anywhere or do anything without paying for it with lost energy. Forget exercise, even a ten-minute walk down the lane wears her out.

She doesn't know when she will see her daughter. She can't handle the drive, and her daughter works so hard and doesn't get much time off.

Nick couldn't understand why she wasn't getting better. He was raised in a farming family that ignored illness and ignored emotions. He was uncomfortable with her chronic complaints. He just wanted her to take a few drugs, snap out of it, and help out with the home chores and mowing, duties he expected of a farm wife. He gets frustrated, and Lori was upset that he just didn't understand.

The stepchildren she inherited with her marriage were the products of the dysfunctional relationships of a broken family. They were uncomfortable with Lori, and their response was to ignore her at family events. Her mother-in-law was difficult and closer to the ex-wife than to Lori. She felt unloved, unappreciated, alone, and misunderstood.

Lori was ready to do anything to change this situation. We discussed how it was going to take effort on her part to change her health. She needed to change her diet, change her sleeping habits, and take the appropriate nutrients. Her older farm home had some mold that was affecting her as well, so she needed to have that cleaned and repaired. In addition, Lori needed to confront her feelings about her husband, her mother-in-law, and her stepchildren.

I worked with Lori for several years, and it was not an easy road. She was up and down and had periods of improvement, then she would backslide again. However, she never lost hope and continually took actions to improve her health.

We worked on the right nutrients to improve her ability to make energy. I sent out for neurotransmitter testing to see if we could improve her sleep. It was successful, and she sleeps soundly most nights. We examined her DNA and learned that there were weaknesses she inherited related to her ability to make energy and with her immunity. She got regular massage and Reiki treatments.

Gradually, her energy improved, her immunity improved, and she rarely missed work. She was able to drive to and from work and still take her dog for a walk when she got home. Lori is now able to help with the mowing and attend most of the grandchildren's events. She dropped more than thirty-five pounds; her eyes are bright, and her skin is clear. She still looks at her energy as a precious commodity and takes plenty of time to rest and preserve it. If she does too much, she is much quicker in her recovery.

The biggest change I have seen over the time we worked together is her forgiveness of herself and the people in her life. She had wanted her husband and his family to feel sorry for her, to understand her illness and what she was experiencing. The family with its dysfunctions was unable to do this. It took time to acknowledge and understand that it wasn't possible to change them. She had to be okay with the situation and learn not to be triggered by events. She had to release herself from being the victim. She learned that it was not her job and not really her problem to fix their dysfunction. She had to change herself and her attitudes. This is the only thing we have control over, our reactions to the people and situations that we find ourselves in. Yes, she can still be triggered by family, but she has developed strategies to healthily deal with her emotions.

She becomes stronger and more powerful each day. She has washed the swamp clean with better function and better attitudes, just as the rain washed the African Queen free of the swampy reeds. I envy her strength and tenacity. I am reminded to embrace more of my own!

## Nutritional Strategies

The number-one thing I see with people with Pluto challenges and chronic disease, low energy, and autoimmune is an overgrowth of yeast, most often candida, in the body. Yeast overgrowth dramatically lowers the body's ability to make energy by interfering with the production of energy itself. Every kind of living tissue, whether it is a human being or a bacteria or yeast, needs nourishment and it also eliminates. Anyone with constipation problems knows how miserable it can make you feel.

Sugar, the glucose molecule, feeds yeast in the body, and what yeast eliminates interferes with energy production. An overgrowth of yeast is like putting sugar in the gas tank of your vehicle. Nothing I have seen in practice decreases the body's ability to make energy faster than the overgrowth of yeast.

How does yeast overgrowth occur? The most common cause is taking antibiotics. Antibiotics kill off the bacteria in the body, the good and the bad, the drugs cannot distinguish a good bacterium from a bad one. This leaves an environment where the bacteria are gone, and the yeast that lives there fills in the space. We hear of women needing to take products for vaginal yeast infections all the time after taking antibiotics, though the yeast is not only in the vaginal area. Yeast becomes systemic, causing havoc throughout the body.

Another challenge is that antibiotics deplete the number of mitochondria in cells. So taking antibiotics is a double whammy as far as energy production is concerned. With less mitochondria, the ones left don't function as well due to yeast interfering with energy production. A person who already has low energy due to genetic factors or other health challenges can take a long time to recover from a round of antibiotics.

Other causes of yeast overgrowth include corticosteroid use, diabetes, and just simply flooding the body with too much sugar. The "average" American ingests about 150 pounds of sugar per year by consuming sugary snacks and sodas, higher than any other country.[40]

Some drugs can decrease yeast in the body, but they are hard on the liver. However, numerous natural antifungal, anti-yeast, formulations are very effective.

In addition to taking natural antifungal supplements, limit sugars as much as possible. I have my patients follow a yeast-clearing diet that limits the ingestion of all foods that will raise blood sugar quickly, including but not limited to all sugars, fruits, fruit juices, breads, and other foods made from grains, potatoes, peanuts and peanut butters, and vinegars. Low-sugar vegetables, lean meats, and good fats for a period, two or three weeks, combined with anti-fungal supplements and nutrients will support immunity.

This change alone can be the major metamorphosis required to begin a healing journey. Sugar is very addictive and a real challenge to give up. I have had numerous patients unable or unwilling to release sugar from the diet for even a short time.

Probiotics to replenish the good bugs in the digestive tract are helpful, especially if the person has a history of antibiotic or corticosteroid use, or if treating the yeast overgrowth in the body. Multiple patients have reported nipping colds and flus in the bud with extra probiotics. If you have enough "good bugs" in the gut, the "bad bugs" can only come for a visit!

Gut flora, known as the microbiome, are the yeasts, bacteria, and viruses that live in the digestive tract. We need a healthy microbiome to protect and defend and make some of our necessary nutrients.

These organisms in the digestive tract, when out of equilibrium, allow an environment internally where digestion is disturbed, immune system is compromised, and diseases can occur. An irritated, imbalanced microbiome can adversely affect mental health. This imbalance can also cause illness after a person has taken certain medications. If the digestive tract has been disturbed by antibiotics, birth control pills, prednisone, or other medications that interfere with the good bugs that live in the digestive tract, then the person has imbalanced gut flora, and diminished immune system function. We need them and want them to live in harmony with us, happy and in balance. Replenish them with probiotics.

## Creative Visualization

Travel in your mind until you are sitting by a body of water. Visualize releasing all that no longer serves you into the water. Allow yourself enough time to grieve what you are leaving behind. As change occurs, it is okay to grieve.

## Emotional Strategies

Get supportive help, such as neuro-coaching or cognitive behavioral therapy, to get the help you require for your well-being especially if emotions feel overwhelming, or if strategies to deal with trauma or emotions are needed.

## Relationship Strategies

Review your childhood and the significant events that shaped your life. Are there painful events that occurred prior to your ability to cognitively process what was happening? Are you still triggered by these events? What are the lessons learned from these events? Work with a professional if frequently triggered by these memories or if help is required to move beyond automatic responses to life events.

## Environmental Strategies

Avoid toxic molds and funguses as much as possible. People have developed serious health conditions including brain changes. If exposed, use protective gear to clear the area or hire professionals to clean it for you.

Parasites are prevalent in society. Indications of a possible parasitic infection include unexplained skin rashes, anal itching, chronic digestive issues. If traveling to foreign countries, watch for eating raw fish or undercooked pork. Other parasites are carried by insects or animals. Work with a functional health practitioner to explore natural ways to eliminate parasites and to build immunity so you are not so susceptible.

## Physical Strategies

Lymphatic drainage techniques performed by a physical therapist or a massage therapist are helpful as well as putting your feet up the wall.

In addition to injuries, the musculoskeletal system is frequently an indicator of internal problems. I have often seen shoulder problems and pain in the shoulder blades, indicating a digestive problem or a heart problem. A kidney stone will cause intense splinting of lower back and flank muscles. Lower back, sacroiliac, and hip joints may tell the story of an unhappy colon or an unhappy prostate.

## Mental Strategies

Write out lists of pros and cons related to specific conflicts. Explore why you are resistant to changing a habit, eating more healthfully, resisting exercise, or healing a relationship.

## Genetic Strategies

Pluto energy is related to our cells and the genetic material found within. Ancestral patterns of hurt, betrayal, sadism, manipulation of others, self-destruction and addiction, revenge, and mass murder, such as the holocaust, can be carried over to multiple generations. The energy of these negative patterns is carried to us through our DNA. It is up to each individual to first recognize the patterns and then figure out how to release or transmute the energy to healthier expression.

Recognition that patterns can be generational (i.e. family histories of abuse, alcoholism, and depression) can bring the light of healing to these patterns and heal your entire lineage moving forward. Working with a practitioner who specializes in optimizing genetic function can be helpful to shift and change these ancestral emotional patterns.

Perhaps genetics are why some children and babies get cancer. While it is sad, it is also impossible to know with certainty since environmental factors and inherited genetics can predispose one to cancer as well.

# NEPTUNE

## TRUST INTERCONNECTION

### Associated Body Parts

feet

### Associated Symptoms and Diseases

Alzheimer's and other dementias
addictions
psychosis

The shaman had asked us to imagine lying in the sand, feeling the crash of waves landing on my body. I laid on the floor, visualizing the power of the surf on my body. My imagination allowed the current to carry me out, deep into the ocean. I could feel myself immersed in the depths. I could see neon fish as they darted in and out of the nearby reef and through the mossy green and hazelnut-brown seaweed moving slowly and softly, back and forth with the current.

Flowing, a gentle rocking as the currents move me soothingly beneath the waves. I feel a deep connection with the ocean, my water, the ocean's water, all one.

It reminds me of Indra's net with pearls that reflect all the other pearls as described in Buddhist philosophy, or this quote by Alan Watts describing his interpretation of the same thing: "Imagine a multidimensional spider web in the early morning, covered with dew drops. And every dew drop contains the reflection of all the other dew drops. And, in each reflected dew drop, the reflections of all the other dew drops in that reflection. And so ad infinitum. That is the Buddhist conception of the universe in an image."

The ocean and this sense of connection and oneness is the image and feeling of the astrological archetype of Neptune. We are all linked in ways we don't understand and don't need to.

All healing occurs via the universal intelligence that knows just what to do. The body has an innate ability to heal itself, and it continues to do so as long as we are here. This is the power of universal intelligence represented here as Neptune energy.

Many of us think of the body as something separate from us; we disconnect from it. We even talk about it as something apart from us or as an enemy. I chuckle when I think of the men who describe their pain as feminine and separate from them: "This leg, she's really acting up today," or "I wish you could just cut it off this arm, she's keeping me awake."

Yet we are all connected. The inside and the outside of the body are united, and we are linked to each other.

I was about seventeen when I first felt that oneness consciousness between myself and the universe as a whole. A friend and I decided to take some psychedelic mushrooms as an experiment, just to see what would happen. I was young, wild, and adventurous, ready for anything and impervious to risk and danger, as so many young people are. I also had low self-esteem, didn't want to be left out, and wanted to be accepted by my friends.

After the night of a late-season winter storm in mid-April, we went out in the morning to see sparkling snow on every surface. The colors were brighter, the sun twinkled, and the sky was a robin's-egg blue. The wet, glimmering snow hung on every tree bough and every telephone line. The cacophony of spring birds flitted about, chirping and tweeting their love songs. The world was so beautiful, my heart expanded; and I felt so much a part of all life. I could feel the bond between myself and that crystalline sparking world, a tiny insignificant piece, yet even that tiny piece felt enormous. Reflections, patterns, and numbers repeat in time and space. On the earth and in the water. Each tiny atom, a reflection of each massive galaxy in the universe.

I can now reach this feeling of connection without the use of drugs, yet I understand the desire to use drugs to escape to this place of beauty and oneness. When there is an imbalance in the Neptune archetypal energy, people want to drift off into that universal consciousness. One can drift away into a world of drug abuse and addiction, checking out of this reality and becoming lost in another. Escaping to a world of brighter colors, enhanced sensation, and once again having a sense of connection, if even for a few moments, and escape the harsh reality of life as we know it.

Addiction to these feelings can be strong, especially in those with DNA markers for increased risk. The brain lights more in some people when these pathways are stimulated in the brain. Society must find ways to make people feel safe, secure, and connected so they don't feel as if they must escape into oblivion with drugs.

Understanding of one's increased risk is a valuable personal awareness, and that is possible with genetic technology. We can impact those propensities with lifestyle changes and nutrients, and the environment plays a role.

We can use earth energy to balance Neptune's water energy. Get grounded. Simply put your feet directly on the earth. Smell some flowers. Watch the birds. In winter where it is cold, place your back against a tree. Feel your own roots sinking deep into the earth and connecting with the earth's molten core. Plant some flowers and feel the energy of this earth teeming with life as the hands get dirty and the feet sink deep into the moist soil. If you enjoy gardening, plant some vegetables, and watch them grow just for you. Feel your connection to the planet that sustains us. Observe the seasons and the times of the day.

I planted tulips, knowing that winter was approaching, yet trusting in spring with its emerging beauty bursting forth from the earth with Mars energy. Hug a tree or have a meaningful conversation, staying present in the moment, instead of drifting off into deep waters of oblivion.

Develop a deep trust in the spiritual world and know that everyone is part of it. Maybe then each of us will want to stay here, stay present, feeling oneness on the conscious level together. Appreciating the moments of life and observing the world with our emotions and senses is truly magical.

> "Magic is an emotion that someone feels when they witness something amazing. It could be a shared experience, which is what I try to make my magic about. I want it to be an experience that we shared together."
>
> —Dynamo

Some people escape permanently to this place, long before death, with Alzheimer's or other forms of dementia. This is an escape into a childlike world, checking out early from parts of life, perhaps getting lost along the way.

My grandmother, Beatrice, had dementia, though no one called it that then. They called it "hardening of the arteries." My mother recognized that her mother was slipping away, and she was placed in the position of making the tough decisions about her parents.

Grandma was six-feet tall with gray hair, and a long, almost hooked nose. She sat staring blankly out the front window, down the lane of her farmhouse. She rocked and rocked in her wooden rocking chair, looking through her thick lenses at the corn fields, the house sparrows and chickadees, the little creek winding through, and the distant road, with her deep-blue eyes.

In earlier days, if a person had cataracts removed, they didn't replace the lens in the eye but gave individuals super-thick glasses to replace the lens. The thick lenses made her eyes appear considerably larger, which fascinated a younger me.

She lived alone on the farm for the ten years since my grandpa died. Since she lived alone, she had stopped preparing regular meals. Mom eventually discovered that Grandma had stopped eating almost everything except oatmeal.

Mom brought Grandma home to our house for about a month, but it soon became clear that she couldn't stay with us. She was conversing with her parents, long dead, and sister Pearl, left behind in Maryland years before, when she was a teenager moving to Illinois.

That wasn't so bad until she started using our oven like a woodstove, throwing in burning paper or tissues to try to light the stove. It became apparent that she was a danger to herself and the whole family. My mother and her siblings made a difficult decision to put her into a nursing home.

Within a year, Grandma was unable to recognize any family members. I went to see her, but it was so difficult for me, a sensitive teenager, not to be recognized. She always seemed happy when we went to visit her. Her face lit up with a smile if I gave her a hug, even if she didn't know who I was. She lived like this for more than ten years, childlike and constantly cared for.

Beatrice had escaped into her own world, a world with no responsibility and no stress. Her soul retreated to its origin, checking out early.

Is there a way to prevent Alzheimer's? This question is scrutinized daily, and research is underway.

I don't believe there is a magic pill that will fix dementia problems. Yes, my Grandma Bea's diet was horrible, and I am certain it was a contributing factor. Research has linked insulin resistance and blood sugar handling to dementia. Some are now calling dementia "diabetes type-III." My family's genetics show huge tendencies toward blood sugar dysregulation.

Blood sugar regulation, keeping our brains active, exercise, and optimizing genetic function by plugging in nutrients to overcome inherited weakness are what we can do right now, since these actions are showing promise in prevention, but there is more to research. A 2020 paper published in the journal, *Psychological Science,* showed that people who were generally more cheerful and enthusiastic were less likely to suffer steep memory decline later in life.[41] This propensity to experience positive emotions is known as "positive affect" in psychology. The national study tracked 991 middle-aged-to-older US adults over three time periods, ten years apart from each other. Each study assessed a range of positive emotions that the participants had experienced over the course of thirty days. The final assessment also tested the participants' memory by asking them to recall words immediately after a presentation and then again fifteen minutes later.

Results were measured by analyzing the relationship between positive affect and memory decline, taking into account such things as age, gender, education, depression, negative affect, and extraversion. The researchers found that, although memory consistently declined with age, ". . . individuals with higher levels of positive affect had a less-steep memory decline over the course of almost a decade," as stated by lead author Dr. Emily Hittner, a PhD from Northwestern University.

My invitation is to begin to look at the world with childlike wonder. See the world as a child and get excited with each tiny morsel of divine beauty that is our planet. This is the true prevention. We started this chapter discussing the inner tasks associated with the moon. This expands on the moon task of nurturing the inner child.

I remember gazing at my one-year-old granddaughter and sensing her delight at the smallest things. One day she was meowing out the window and waving at a kitty through the screen door. Pay attention to the children in your life, and watch how they look at the world and how they play. You can play too!

Play more, dance more, and find joy in each moment. Smell the flowers, laugh more, and get more hugs. Be silly and have fun!

## Nutrient Strategies

The truth is that we live in a buggy world. We need the bugs, yeasts, fungus, bacteria, worms, insects, and spiders in our external environments and yeasts, fungus, and bacteria in our internal environments. The symbiotic relationship with these bugs is an important component to our health and well-being.

The healthy bacteria in our digestive tracts protect us from the more dangerous bugs that cause infections. If we have enough good bugs, then bad bugs can only come for a visit. In fact, small amounts of staph and strep bacteria live in our bodies all the time. They are not a concern if the immune system, digestive tract, and bowel are balanced.

Unfortunately, as mentioned earlier, antibiotics, birth control pills, cortisone-type medication, and other medications cause an imbalance in the normal digestive bacteria, or gut flora. The gut flora is also upset and imbalanced by stress and by too much sugar in the diet.

In addition to taking probiotics, people can eat foods with natural bacteria that will populate the digestive tract with healthy organisms. This is what our ancestors used for probiotics. Fermented foods like sauerkraut, kimchi, kombucha, or sourdough bread will add healthy bacteria, along with eating cultured yogurts or cheeses (if your body does well with fermented foods or dairy). Genetic testing will show if you are able to handle large amounts of these types of foods.

Foods high in fiber work as prebiotics, creating the healthy environment and nourishment that promote the growth of good bugs or probiotics. Examples of high fiber foods include artichokes, radishes, carrots, cucumbers, beets, sweet potato, yams, garlic, onions, chicory root, and cabbage, to name a few.

## Creative Visualization

Using your imagination, explore and create a world of delight using all your senses. Notice how your bodily sensations create the conditions for your soul and consciousness to feel at home. Visualize bringing this world fully into consciousness.

## Emotional Strategies

Neptune is where you want to look at the whole picture, to expand and get a worldview. What will create balance, synergy, and a feeling of wholeness within? What will work for you?

Many times, it is as simple as choosing how to react to the events in life rather than simply reacting. Just stopping for a moment and deciding. Something is happening. I am feeling a reaction. What can I do?

Yawn deeply, mouth open, and stretch with arms extended like on arising. Follow by rubbing both hands together sensuously if that is comfortable for you. Being sensuous requires being in the moment. Thoughts can't be lost somewhere else, in the past or in the future. This sensuous activity brings you back to this moment. This moment is the only place to make a decision about what it is and how you are going to react to what life is hurling at you.

## Relationship Strategies

Other times, we need the help and support of others to help us to find our way out of anxiety, depression, PTSD, or other mental health problems. Medications may be required, at least for a time, but medications are not the only answers. Many answers can be found in finding the right nutrients to turn happy brain patterns by stimulating areas of the brain that improve mood and feelings of well-being.

Spending time with friends and family can be life sustaining and nurturing to the soul, and it can also extend life. Be certain to carve out time on a regular basis to spend with people who are closest to you.

## Environmental Strategies

Eat organic and drink pure water. Avoid exposure to large amounts of herbicides and pesticides in foods and water, which means eating organic as much as possible and purifying water of chemicals. Eat minimally processed, real foods as often as possible.

Consider water filters to additionally purify the water you drink to limit your exposure to chlorine, fluoride, and other chemicals and toxins that interfere with the hormones that travel through your bloodstream and lymphatics.

## Physical Strategies

Childlike activities and play are the best way to get Neptune energies flowing. Can you recall the specific things or can you recreate the feelings? It does matter! Create time for play. Remember what you loved doing at age ten? Can you do the same things? Can you make modifications and still have fun? Play, play a lot, play some more! If you don't know how to play, ask for help with play therapy.

## Mental Strategies

Get very clear about what you don't want in life.

What is it you want to move away from? What will life be like if I do nothing?

Five years from now? Ten years from now? What will life be and how will it feel?

This process helps to gain clarity about what you do want. I find it also helps to focus on the feelings that you want to have moving into the future.

## Genetic Strategies

Research continues to demonstrate that thoughts, movement, environment, and foods all impact genetic expression. Decide to impact genetic function positively by being optimistic, moving frequently, limiting exposure to toxins as much as possible, and eating real food, including lots of plants.

I invite you to create a personal path to health and well-being. What works for me doesn't work for someone else. Each person has to find their own path to well-being and health. Each one learns to trust the body's messages, and each person needs to find their place in this amazing world. Take everything in. Don't dismiss anything. Even negative emotions—allow them to be felt. However, don't leave negative emotions stuck inside. Sort out what triggered the emotion and what you can do about it. Think of the inside as the garden where you plant the seeds of thoughts and emotion. A healthy garden is mulched with healthy soil and compost teeming with life and allowing for growth. A healthy body will do the same. Turn ideas and emotions around and share outwardly with the world.

We are all connected. We are all in this world together. Observe the interconnections, and they become more apparent.

## CHAPTER SEVEN
# AIR ARCHETYPES

## Air

We often forget about the air that surrounds us because it is invisible, unless of course you live where there is lots of smog and pollution held within the air. Yet we recognize its intense power when we hear of windstorms, tornados, and hurricanes, and the path of destruction that so often accompanies powerful winds.

The air around us, when unpolluted, is perfect for life. It combines a variety of gasses: primarily nitrogen and oxygen, with almost 1 percent argon, and even smaller amounts of carbon dioxide and other elements such as krypton and helium.

Air works in harmony with the trees and plants on the planet that provide the oxygen we need to breathe, manufactured by photosynthesis in green leaves. We provide the carbon dioxide in our exhalations.

The water in the ocean plays a huge role in this intricate dance of life, as it produces over half of the world's oxygen and absorbs fifty times more carbon dioxide than our atmosphere. Air carries water and the water vapor warms our planet, and rain sustains the life of the plants and animals on the earth.

Air does have mass, has volume, and it exerts pressure. Just try pushing a beach ball to the bottom of a swimming pool and see if it stays there. The air compressed by the water needs to find more space and pops to the surface. Air is actually a force that pushes down on us constantly, however our bodies also exert a pressure that balances the external pressure of the air outside.

We require the oxygen carried in the air to provide the oxygen for our blood that carries that basic building block, oxygen, to all the parts of the body. Oxygen is part of protein and carbohydrate metabolism, required for building new cells, making energy, feeding the brain, and supporting immunity. Every cell Every cell "breaths" through through a process called cellular respiration, where we combine oxygen with a variety of molecules for life-sustaining actions and discarding waste products, carbon dioxide, and water.

Air carries sound and is in constant motion. Our society talks of "the winds of change" and "fanning the flames." Air lifts invisible particles and moves molecules.

The three air archetypes are Mercury of Gemini, Venus of Libra, and Uranus of Aquarius. Words that express the energy of air include; contact, connection, openness, harmony, curiosity, spontaneous, idealism, communication, innovation, balance, originality, social, collaboration, and partnership. Others with out-of-balance air can be liars, opportunistic, sensationalist, gossiping, vain, indecisive, maniac, rebels, and anarchists.

We begin with Mercury of Gemini.

## MERCURY OF GEMINI

## COMMUNICATION AND CONNECTION

### Associated Body Parts

>   lungs
>   circulatory system
>   circulating hormones
>   nerves and neurotransmitters
>   hands

### Associated Symptoms and Diseases

>   bronchitis
>   bronchial cancer
>   lung embolism
>   pneumonia
>   emphysema
>   asthma
>   circulation diseases
>   diseases of the nervous system

This was a story told to me by a friend.

Nancy was my best friend when I was a little girl. We played with Barbie dolls and we danced in the hot summer sun while her big sister's 45-vinyl records played on a small portable record player outside of her dad's garage. We were neighbors, and I could see her house just across the cul-de-sac from where we lived.

On lazy summer days, we stealthily crept into the kitchens of our homes and sneaked cookies, crackers, cheese slices, cans of tuna, and bags of chips, and took them on adventures with us as we explored new houses under construction on the new streets nearby. Our neighborhood was ever-expanding during the late sixties and seventies when we were growing up. I am sure our moms were aware of what we were pilfering, but we thought we were getting away with something.

Nancy was petite and had long, blonde hair. I was younger by a year, and taller, never petite, with dark-brown hair. I always envied her beautiful suntan, while I struggled with freckles and sunburn.

She was the outgoing one, always ready for the next adventure. I was drawn to her because I was terribly shy, and outgoing Nancy loved to talk with anyone and everyone. I was as adventurous and ready to tag along, even though I often hung back and watched.

Nancy and I drifted apart, as children do when they go off in different directions and different interests. Since she was a year older than me, we didn't hang out together at school. She was never very intellectual, and academics were not her forte, while I was driven by a family dynamic to achieve higher grades and to excel at school. She was loving, kind, and fiercely loyal.

We stayed in touch over the years as we drifted in and out of each other's lives. We seemed to reach out to each other during momentous occasions, births, graduations, weddings, deaths, or in times of crisis. Otherwise, we lived separate lives in different communities.

Nancy was one of those people to whom all that was required for a conversation was to say hello and goodbye. After that the conversation took on a life of its own. It was possible to squeeze in a question from time to time, if you were lucky. Nancy filled in the rest.

She was not the person to share a secret with. It would be asking too much for her to hold it in. She was the person to share news with if you wanted all your friends and acquaintances to be aware. Meaningful conversations were challenging. Her stories were like social media posts; gossip, news snippets, school friends, and celebrity stories. She would puff on a cigarette and talk and talk.

Nancy had always dreamed of moving to the Rocky Mountains. She had lived there as a young woman and always wished and dreamed of retirement living high in the mountains. She yearned to be close to her son, brother, and other family who lived there.

Every time I visited Nancy, the talk included moving to Montana. She was going to buy a large camper and live in it during retirement. Her husband Max was going to retire early, and they were going to move.

In Nancy's situation, this was a pipe dream. She was powerless in many ways, and had no ability to make it happen.

I quit smoking thirty years ago, and she continued to smoke most of her life. Nancy developed severe lung conditions; emphysema, eventual lung disease, and lung failure. She and her husband Max were both smokers.

She worked hard at several different jobs in her lifetime but never had much money of her own. Max had a steady job, yet the money went out faster than it came in. She often said she wanted to come to visit me at my home but had to stay home because her car was falling apart, or there wasn't money for gas to make the eighty-mile trek.

Her home was a small two-bedroom bungalow that further deteriorated each time I visited over the thirty years she lived there. The brown shag carpet grew increasingly threadbare and faded, and the floor became squishy and gave way a bit with each step. There was dust on the surfaces and dirt in the corners. The house reeked of tobacco. Nancy said she quit smoking, but she still had to have a puff now and then. All the extra money had been going to pay for cigarettes and, toward the end, the medical bills to keep her alive.

The last time she went to the mountains to visit her brother and son who lived in Montana, she could hardly breathe and had to return home early. It required a trip to the hospital and weeks to recover.

Near the end of her life, Nancy's son called to ask if I would be willing to spend his wedding day with his mom. Nancy's lung condition had gotten so bad she was unable to travel to the mountains to be at her son's wedding. Travel and mountain air would likely have killed her.

I arrived at her home on the wedding day, and we hugged. Nancy chatted away in a very weak breathy way, grappling for air as she told me about the wedding preparations and the rest of the family in Montana. Her nose held the long tubing to the flow of oxygen she now needed constantly. Stoic and resigned, Nancy held her emotions in check, holding back tears while telling me, "It's all right," in a rough and scratchy voice.

Nancy looked puffy and had a round face so commonly associated with chronic steroid use. That face held only a glimpse of the beauty she once was. Years of prednisone and struggling for breath had left its mark.

Her son had left instructions to watch a specific DVD he sent at the time of the wedding, which turned out to be a beautiful wedding video with panoramic views of the Rocky Mountains. Nancy could see her handsome son standing in his tux along with her new daughter-in-law dressed in a wedding dress, standing with him, a breathtaking view surrounding them.

We let the tears flow as we watched the video together. She was a good mom; so proud of her son, and she loved him dearly. It broke my heart to watch her suffer. So difficult to watch Nancy's son living out her mother's dream, knowing that now her own dream would never be fulfilled, knowing that she would be left behind. She passed away at home less than a year later. Nancy was not yet sixty.

This story speaks of Mercury. Mercury energy has to do with information overload. Our world is filled with examples of this overload with computers, cellphones, and hundreds of TV channels to spend time surfing through. Power lines, cell towers, and highways twelve lanes across are the feeling and energy of Mercury. Congestion, traffic lights, stores stuffed with overpriced, cheap merchandise imported from Asia also represent Mercury's energy. It is hard to make decisions with so much information and so many choices coming at us. It is hard to separate the trivial from the significant.

Lungs relate to communication. There is no speaking without air. In clinical practice, I see that lungs are often affected when there is grief, sadness, yearning, cloudy thinking, anguish, sorrow, or sudden death, fear of death, or a close call related to death.

Linda is another major talker, extremely difficult to get the words in edgewise. I struggle to get off the phone when she calls, or to get out of the treatment room when she visits the office. Her Mercury imbalance shows up as varicose veins, and we have taken some pressure off those by supporting lymphatic drainage with some nutrients. She is at least aware that she talks too much but doesn't yet feel inclined to change the habit.

I have really worked on my own communication skills. Shy as a child and young adult, and intimidated by my physical body's response of intense blushing when I was unsure of my words, I held things in and did not speak up. I didn't trust or want to communicate in writing, because I held trauma from being chastised about my writing early on.

My choices have moved me far away from that shy intimidated little girl. I became a doctor where I would spend my working life communicating with patients so they could make healthcare choices and understand their bodies better. I have been running businesses where I had to learn the balance between giving to others, listening to others, and taking enough time for myself. I learned business management, letting staff be heard, and let them understand what I need for support.

I had to learn to have more genuine communication, releasing my fears of showing my authentic self. I have grown in my ability to speak up for myself and my own needs and to hear the needs of others more clearly.

One powerful learning was to create more balance in my communication by asking permission more often before offering my opinion or advice. My ingrained habit was to automatically tell people what they should do for their health. I still catch myself doing that, but it is becoming less frequent. Writing this book is also an attempt to overcome my hurdle related to writing, and to create new dimensions in my communication skills.

Each person desires to be seen and heard. We all face challenges and conflict in communication. Communication is a work in progress, always in flux. One conversation is clear and easy, and the next can make us angry or frustrated. Communication expands our connection to others, just as a road trip takes us to our friend's home, an electric wire brings electricity to a lamp, or an online meeting connects each one to a business conference.

Take a moment and celebrate the magic of all the communication carried out in the physical body. The body has input from all our senses. Messages are carried via nerves and molecules in blood to individual tissues and cells. Truly miraculous! Take a moment to feel gratitude and appreciation for the miracle the body is, and for all the ways it communicates.

In the body, when communication works well, the nervous system and hormonal systems work in harmony. The hypothalamus, the part of the brain that communicates with the hormonal system, communicates with the pituitary gland and vice versa. The pituitary gland sends messages to all the other organs that produce hormones via the circulatory system; the thyroid, the pancreas, the stomach, ovaries or testes, and even body fat receives the messages.

Body fat produces multiple hormones that work in balance with all the others when functioning properly. Here are just a few found in fat:[42]

- leptin (1994) regulates appetite;
- adiponectin (1995) increases insulin sensitivity, reduces inflammation;
- ADAMTS1 (1997) influences fat stem cell differentiation, blood vessel formation, ovulation;

- chemerin (1997) increases inflammation, raises blood pressure;
- resistin (2001) mediates resistance to insulin;
- retinol-binding protein 4 (2005) is implicated in insulin resistance;
- lipocalin-2 (2007) increases insulin resistance and inflammation;
- isthmin-1 (2014) improves fat metabolism in the liver, mediates immune system, influences developmental patterning;
- asprosin (2016) modulates glucose release from the liver;
- Slit2-C (2016) spurs glucose metabolism; and
- lipocalin-5 (2018) enhances skeletal muscle respiration.

I think of the interplay between the hormones as a dance that can be perfectly choreographed like a pair of ballroom dancers performing a waltz, or the frenetic head-banging, body slamming dance of a heavy metal concert. Stress is the primary factor that throws the dance into a frenzy.

Lezley has four children, ages six years and younger. She came in with all the children, baby seat, and diaper bag in tow. She was still nursing the youngest at ten months. Lezley, five-foot-seven and 134 pounds, was tired and having lots of digestive trouble. Her rest was often disturbed by one or more of the children. Her last pregnancy was really tough with a great deal of morning sickness. She had tried lots of different supplements, in fact she brought in an entire bag full of products, but was still having bloating and indigestion almost constantly. Her husband had a very busy job that kept him away for ten hours or more a day and often had evening meetings as well, so she often felt stuck at home with the busy job of mothering.

Her examination revealed that she was borderline anemic, a deficiency in iron, causing a decrease in the carrying capacity of her red blood cells to get oxygen to her cells. This was why she was exhausted. She was also deficient in other minerals, calcium and magnesium especially, and essential fatty acids necessary to form healthy cell membranes and keep inflammation reduced. Quite likely her body was depleted due to her numerous pregnancies over such a short period. Fetuses get all the nutrients they need in the womb, often leaving mothers depleted.

On evaluation, Lezley required some adrenal gland support to handle the stress of her daily life, and pituitary support to get all the hormones working together in harmony. Within three months, Lezley was feeling much better and had better energy. She was digesting better, and the bloating had stopped. Her sleep was still disturbed by the children, but she still woke more rested in the morning.

We talked about her desire for more self-care and for personal time away from the children. I suggested she hire a sitter or communicate with her husband about ways to make that work for their busy schedules. She loves being a mom and having the opportunity to be home with the children, but she does occasionally need a break. She talked with her husband and now takes a few hours every Saturday to get out of the house. Even though getting out usually entails a trip to the grocery store, at least she gets to go alone.

Four months into our treatment, Lezley was pregnant again. I followed her throughout the pregnancy and the time flew with little discomfort. She now has a beautiful baby boy, and she came out of this pregnancy with ease.

## Nutritional Strategies

Essential means that the body absolutely must have it and, in the case of essential fatty acids, that means we absolutely need them from our diet. The body cannot make essential fatty acids. The essential fats are omega-3 (alpha linolenic acid) and omega-6 (linoleic acid) fats. Every single membrane in the body and every single cell has essential fats. Many of these essential fats are destroyed in the processing of foods. Some fats are converted by heat to trans fats, hydrogenated oils, which increase inflammation and decrease membrane flexibility.

People in generations past had a higher percentage of omega-3 fats when raised farm animals ate the grasses and foraged items in the barnyard or pasture. Modern farming methods have moved enormous numbers of animals into confinement buildings where they are fed primarily corn and soy products, both naturally high in pro-inflammatory omega-6 fats. Cows may begin life in the pasture, but they are often "finished" by adding larger amounts of corn and soy feeds to add weight to the animals and the "marbling" of fat into the meat. The combination of having processed and heated oils and more meats produced by animals in confinement has caused an imbalance in the omega-3 and 6 balance in human bodies resulting in greater inflammation and pain for many.

Omega-3 fats in higher amounts are found in flaxseed, chia seed, walnuts, and mostly in different kinds of fish. Deep-ocean, wild-caught fish have the highest percentage of omega-3 fats. Eating fish at least twice per week is recommended. Vegetarians will want to pay close attention to getting enough of the nuts and seeds to keep fats in balance, sometimes a challenge.

Two types of omega-3 fat are found in fish; EPA (eicosapentaenoic acid) and DHA (docosahexaenoic acid). These highly unsaturated, flexible fatty acids increase flexibility of membranes and improve communication between cells. Both types decrease inflammation, and lower LDL cholesterol. EPA decreases platelet aggregation, a risk factor in heart disease. DHA is vital for infant brain development and adult brain/nerve function. Deficiencies of DHA are associated with, but not limited to, ADHD, dyslexia, depression, aggression, and cognitive impairment.

Health benefits have been seen for chronic pain and swelling, inflammation, immunoregulation, disc herniation, osteoarthritis, autoimmune conditions, diabetes and insulin sensitivity, cardiovascular conditions, asthma and allergies, dermatitis, and kidney problems. I frequently suggest adding fish oil supplementation and even suggest taking a large dosage for a few days rather than reaching for over-the-counter pain medications.

Not all fish oil is created equally. Know the sources and where it is produced to make sure that the raw materials have been tested for heavy metals. Fish often have mercury contamination, a consequence of pollution. Read the labels. Often a label will say "a proprietary blend of fish oil" but doesn't break down the amounts of EPA and DHA. It just says 1,000 mg of fish oil, but that 1,000 mg may only have 20 mg of EPA and even less of DHA. Look to get at least 300 mg of EPA and 200 mg of DHA in 1,000 mg or more.

Be aware that farm-raised fish are often given feed produced from corn and soy as well, so they can even have a higher percentage of omega-6, proinflammatory fat than beef! Choose the deep ocean, wild-caught fish wherever possible.

Frequently a person needs to add additional fish oil, but some require the addition of a balanced formulation with some of the anti-inflammatory omega-6 fats derived from borage oil or evening primrose oil. Menstruating women or girls at menarche, the onset of periods, often require the balance of oils, because both are required to form healthy prostaglandins, hormone-like substances that participate in a wide range of body functions such as the contraction and relaxation of smooth muscle, the dilation and constriction of blood vessels, control of blood pressure, and modulation of inflammation, all-important considerations when having menstrual pain or cramping.

## Creative Visualization

Our world is noisy and busy, which can result in an overload of information. Call upon air and the winds when you want to quiet the noise and communicate clearly and effectively.

Winds can carry desires on its wings and help to fulfill dreams. The wind can also help to find the words to express what is held in the heart.

Air will help you to hear the messages from the Divine more clearly, and the messages and communications you want to share will be carried on the winds with ease and grace.

## Emotional Strategies

People pleasing is seeking acceptance and love from external sources. Shift the focus to the divine feminine core to build self-love, self-acceptance, self-understanding, self-compassion, setting boundaries, and being authentic.

Practice active listening, deeply empathetic listening. The more you learn of others the more you learn about yourself.

## Relationship Strategies

A focus on others stimulates a happier brain, e.g., I am so grateful I could help Mary put away her groceries, or I am so grateful I could help Mark paint the living room at his house.

## Environmental Strategies

Use cleaning products carefully. Use safe home cleaning supplies for cleaning and air freshening. Restrict use of bleach and ammonia products known to damage lung tissue.[43] Many other chemicals are toxic, damage the brain, the eyes, and the liver, and can cause multiple health problems, especially if one has health problems already, or the body doesn't detoxify well. Switch to nontoxic cleaning products whenever possible. Go to EWG.org for a detailed list of safe products in self and home care.

## Physical Strategies

Breathwork is using specific types of breathing to move energy in the body. Breath is the foundation for greater well-being and using breathwork is an art and science to unlock the most correct ways to breathe in any circumstance.

## Mental Strategies

Brainstorm with a group to get new ideas for conflicts, challenges, or ways to grow yourself. No idea is bad!

Get out of stuck habits and enhance brain function by doing things in different ways, e.g. drive to work a different way, brush your teeth with the opposite hand, sit in a different place when eating. This expands your awareness of self and of your environment.

## Genetic Strategies

I love the fact that genes can be impacted in healthy and constructive ways by adding specific nutrients, changing the diet as needed, increasing exercise and healthy movement, and by positive thought and healthy touch.

## VENUS OF LIBRA:

## CREATING SENSUALITY AND APPRECIATING BEAUTY

### Associated Body Parts

skin as a sensual contact organ
pancreas
kidneys

### Associated Symptoms and Diseases

kidney disease, acute and chronic
glomerulonephritis
polycystic kidney disease
urinary tract infections
hypoglycemia
diabetes
acne
atopic dermatitis (eczema)
shingles (herpes zoster)
herpes, simplex 1 and 2
hives (urticaria)
sunburn
contact dermatitis
rosacea
warts
ringworm
impetigo

Ruth, an executive in charge of more than fifty employees, came to see me for right leg and ankle swelling. She reported it came on gradually over the previous three months. It wasn't painful, but she was quite concerned. Her ankle was puffy, and her shoe was tight. My body scan revealed that her right kidney was the primary problem. The kidneys, related to Venus of Libra, the archetype associated with balance and sensuality.

Imagine walking through the Louvre museum in Paris, admiring the statues and the fine art, then taking the train to Versailles where wandering through the palace grounds and perfectly designed gardens is a sensual delight. Feel the exquisite balance of the design, see the extravagance and the ornate beauty. Visualize a princess and the prince strolling among the statues and fountains on the grounds. This sensual appreciation is the essence of Venus of Libra.

Ruth is strikingly beautiful with bright, green eyes and a warm smile. Fifty-four years old, she wears her business suit and chunky-gold matching jewelry. Her makeup is impeccable, and her brown hair is stylishly cut at shoulder length. She is the consummate professional.

In addition to her busy job, she stops by and cares for her elderly parents at the end of each workday. Her siblings live across the country, so the job of checking on mom and dad has fallen to her. She is the oldest daughter, and her two brothers expect her to take the responsibility.

She knows her mom and dad are failing a bit, but for now they are stable and can live at home without assistance. They wouldn't take assistance from anyone outside of the family anyway. She truly enjoys the visit at the end of her busy workday. Unfortunately this means she gets home close to 7:00, and she still needs to prepare a meal.

Our consultation revealed that much of her life was about being of service, giving out until there was little to no time to give to herself. I was able to share that I have experienced the same type of imbalance in my own life. My recommendations included nutrients to support her kidney and to help release fluids naturally, and it was effective after a few weeks.

On a follow-up visit, our conversation arrived at how kidneys are related to balance. With work she was not able to create a balance between her masculine and feminine aspects.

Since it was on the right side, the masculine side, her body was indicating that the masculine side was working too hard in relation to the feminine side. Her job required her to step into a more masculine role by giving instructions to others and by overseeing the office.

I asked her what she could do to enhance her feminine receiving and creative energies. She admitted that she had let her creative juices dry up in the busy-ness of life. Things had gotten out of balance. She assured me that she would take time to rest more and do the things and projects that nurtured her feminine nature.

She pulled out her knitting needles and started baking again. These activities helped her find balance in the past, but she moved these activities to the back burner.

I am not saying that "traditional women's activities" are the only way to nurture. We revealed that nurturing, listening, reflecting, and nurturing creative projects are all feminine in nature. She could very well have chosen to nurture herself with meditation, prayer, and massage. She could have walked in the woods, read a new book, gone to a lecture to hear fresh ideas, listened to music, taken a dance class, or hooked a rug. Ruth chose baking and knitting. Her swelling went away and so did the need for specific nutrients for her kidney.

> "Balance is not something you find. It is something you create."
>
> ~Jana Kingsford

The other major disease related to Venus of Libra and finding balance is diabetes. This time the balance is related to blood sugar.

Of the two types of diabetes, type I, called juvenile diabetes, is when you have an inability to make enough insulin and it appears in childhood. These people must take insulin shots for a lifetime. The second type, type II, is adult-onset diabetes, where diabetes comes on later in life. Unfortunately our society is seeing an increasing number of Type II diabetics who are teenagers.

My family is filled with diabetics, and I have spent a lot of time studying nutritional strategies to balance blood sugar. My maternal grandparents were both diabetic, my mom was a diabetic, and so was my father at the end of his life. My sister and brother are diabetic as well. So far, I have avoided that diagnosis, but I am certain I have insulin resistance. Obviously, there must be a genetic correlation in my family, yet there are many people who develop diabetes with no family history. Diabetes is the fastest-growing and most-expensive disease in our culture. Currently one in three people in the United States have either diabetes or insulin resistance, and that number is expected to increase to one in two over the next decade.

Insulin resistance is when cells can no longer take insulin into the cell. They have too much circulating insulin from eating too much sugar or foods that break down to sugar quickly. It is an early indicator of predisposition to diabetes or associated heart disease. Insulin resistance is like a married couple who have lived together long enough that they tune out their spouse's voice and don't hear what is being said. Like the echo bouncing off the walls of the house, "What did you say?"

Too much circulating insulin causes a person to be in chronic inflammation and to store fat. Left too long, chronic inflammation causes heart disease, neuropathy, diabetes, blindness, increased risk of heart attack and stroke, and early death.

Too much circulating sugar (glucose) is followed by too much circulating insulin, because insulin's job is to get the circulating glucose into cells. When there is too much, the cells simply can't take in anymore glucose or insulin.

Bodies are flooded with sugary beverages, processed cookies and pastries, grains or chips, fruit juices, which all break down to sugar quickly. As mentioned earlier, the average American ingests about 150 pounds of sugar per person each year. We spike our blood sugar multiple times a day with these foods and beverages.

Once you get the diagnosis of Type II diabetes, you have likely been dealing with insulin resistance for ten or more years. Diabetes ages you by fifteen years and is a loss of balance in the glucose levels in the body. Eventually many diabetics, if they poorly manage their diet and don't keep blood sugar regulated, lose their ability to make insulin and need to take insulin shots or have insulin pumps.

Why do we eat so much sugar or foods that break down to sugar quickly?

First, it is readily available, and the food industry is designing ways to entice us to eat processed foods and beverages. Our society has gotten away from cooking meals at home. We watch cooking shows then go to eat large portions at restaurants. One in four children eats a meal per day in a fast-food restaurant.

Second, we are so rushed and frazzled with the pace of life, the need to make money, we forget to stop. We forget to find joy in the moments.

Moments of sweetness go by in a flash, and we fail to feel them. We feel the pain and the frustrations weighing us down and don't notice the sweetness of the hugs we receive or remember eating the cookie. How many times are meals eaten while standing in the kitchen and desserts eaten mindlessly while watching TV?

My extended family, on both sides, experienced generations of poverty, sadness, repeated economic hardships, and hard work from dawn to dusk; sweetness was hard to find. Most people had parents, grandparents, or great-grandparents who lived through the depression, leaving a legacy and genetic blueprint of lack and loss. This heritage may have something to do with the current rise in diabetes in our culture.

I learned something while living on my acreage on the lake. Picking wild raspberries and blackberries is so like life, often it leaves you scratched and injured. Sometimes you have to wear long sleeves, wear protection, even in summer! Yet just as you think you have found all the sweetness and bounty, you turn your head, you get a fresh perspective, and a whole new bunch of sweetness is observed. The sweetness is there, you just have to look for it.

> "Sometimes you will never know the value of a moment until it becomes a memory"
> 
> –Dr. Suess

## Nutritional Strategies

Products that will make you much more sensitive to insulin and will make other systems work better too are magnesium, alpha lipoic acid, chromium, and B-complex. Magnesium, 400 mg daily, and chromium, 200 mcg daily, will improve glycemic response. Alpha-lipoic acid, 600–1,200 mg, will prevent or treat neuropathy. B-complex is important to make cells more sensitive to insulin as well as preventing diabetic complications. It may take additional B6 as pyrodoxyl-5-phosphate, folate as L-5 methyltetrahydrofolate, and B12 as methylcobalamin to get the systems working. Work with a nutritionist to find the right nutrients for you.

## Creative Visualization

Using all your senses, create a clear picture of all that is sweet in your life, whether it be the smile of a child, a beautiful fragrant flower, a warm hug, a picturesque landscape, a deep faith, or a stirring piece of music.

## Emotional Strategies

Mindfulness meditation, even for one minute, helps to be present and notice what is. Combine meditation and mindfulness to focus on the vast expanse of meditation and its importance to healing and health.

Body scan mindfulness meditation may help with relaxation and awareness of different body sensations.

## Relationship Strategies

Review your childhood and the significant events that shaped your life. Are there painful events that occurred prior to your ability to cognitively process what was happening? Are you still triggered by these events? What are the lessons learned from these events?

Work with a professional if frequently triggered by these memories or if help is required to move beyond automatic responses to life events.

## Environmental Strategies

Avoid toxic skin chemicals. Avoiding skin products with toxic chemicals such as parabens, sulfates, phthalates, formaldehyde, phenoxyethanol, to name just a few. Sunscreens can contain chemicals that are toxic as well.

## Physical Strategies

Stimulate Venus of Libra with physically sensual activities, massage, and sex. Even the memory of these activities are an effective way to stimulate the brain and body.

## Mental Strategies

Build internal power with thoughts of validation and worth, prior to a crisis. Brains are wired to look for what is wrong, so actively seek to find what is right.

## Genetic Strategies

Creating perspective and a perception shift will allow life to bring in more sweetness. Paying attention to moments, focusing on gratitude and appreciation, seeing the beauty of nature supports our balance. Drinking in the cornucopia of sensations we experience through our senses is the gift we experience with our bodies. Sensuality and sensuousness in our loving, partnership relationships promote feelings of unity and balance. Observe life and feel life as a precious commodity, filled with beauty, love and harmony. Life offers so much sweetness that we don't need to get it all from our food.

Taste and smell are gifts as well. Savor the moments and the foods you choose to eat. I often tell patients to go ahead and have an occasional dessert, and make sure it's really good! Don't buy a package of cookies and eat them all before paying attention! Enjoy every bite of a single cookie! It will then feed that longing for sweetness without overindulgence.

## URANUS:

## ORIGINALITY, LAUGHTER AND SURPRISE

### Associated Body Parts

ankles

### Associated Symptoms and Diseases

broken bones
sprain/strains
accidents
stroke
myocardial infarction
epilepsy
Tourette's syndrome
tics and twitches
St Vitus dance
stuttering
cramps
attention disorders
panic and fears

The phone rang at 9:00 p.m. It was my dear friend Max sounding anxious and edgy. It was a cold snowy winter night in January. He lives in the Northwest and told me he had just been in a car accident and just needed to talk. He was driving through the mountains and hit black ice on the dark mountain road. The car he was driving skidded and flipped over in the ditch. He was shaken and scared because he had to climb out of the window of the car and climb up out of the ditch.

It was a dark night, and he had to wait by the side of the road for the tow truck and a ride. Fortunately nothing was broken or bleeding. I instructed him to use ice on the injuries to keep the inflammation from escalating, and then we just talked. I also recommended that he seek chiropractic care soon as possible. The car belonged to his partner. They had been living together for five years, and now her car was totaled.

We both needed to talk for a while to calm each other down. The accident had left him shaking and in pain. He needed time and the sound of a friend's voice to melt away the anxiety so he could get to sleep, and I needed to know that he was really okay. I said goodnight to Max after we both felt more relaxed and calmer.

Two weeks later he called me in tears, saying that his partner was leaving him. The relationship was no longer working for her, and she would be leaving soon.

"I don't know what I'm going to do," he cried.

My interpretation is that the signs were there. Accidents often happen when something needs shaking up. Were there problems in the relationship that needed to be addressed? Undoubtedly. This was the beginning of the end, and the accident heralded the breakup. She has now moved on, and he is reinventing his life, finding ways to cope with the new situation.

Accidents, broken bones, stroke, tics, and stutters are examples of how the Uranus energy shows up in the body.

Here is another example of how Uranus energy is observed. Margie continually injured the same right ankle, at least once per year. She was incredibly shy, introverted, fearful, and dreaded going to any large gatherings. When I visited Margie's home, the news was on constantly, and she lived in fear of the world.

In college she met and made friends with three women. They gathered once per year for a weekend get-together. These women were her circle, and they all lived miles away. Other than immediate family, Margie had few other outside relationships. Each year she went to the same location on the same vacation. Once her husband convinced her to be brave, and she traveled to Ireland. She sprained her ankle badly on that trip and had to miss a number of tours.

She was a dear woman, and I loved her; however her life lacked spontaneity, originality, and adventure. She feared the world, and feared showing her unique self to the world. She was a brittle diabetic, meaning she had trouble getting her blood sugars stabilized. The day before she died, she took a tumble, missing a single step and falling. The next day her life ended when she had a sudden heart attack. She was sixty-eight.

Her body was showing her throughout her life that something needed to be shaken up by giving her the repeated sprained ankles. Yet nothing changed. She continued to be timid, apprehensive, and anonymous till the end of her shortened life.

Another example of a life that was shaken up was the life of Jill Bolte Taylor. Her book, *My Stroke of Genius*, tells the story of this neuroscientist who had a major stroke.

Stroke strikes suddenly. Often with devastating results. She tells the story of how she felt experiencing the stroke, knowing what it was. She was trapped in her own brain, understanding what was happening but unable to communicate. It took her eight years to fully recover, but her insights are extraordinary. She says now that she knew that "I was going to be somebody new."

One of her marvelous insights as she healed was to move toward whole brain living. She says she focuses on who she's going to be in each moment.

Along with her science, she now finds that "art is delicious" in a short video I saw put out by AARP, I saw her working on stained glass art, making sun catchers that look like beautiful brains. Her advice, "Keep your brain cells excited."

## Nutritional Strategies

Accidents and injuries require the same nutrients. It is important to get the inflammation down as quickly as possible. Tumeric extract, 200 mg; botswellia extract, 200 mg; ginger extract, 200 mg; and rosemary extract, 50 mg are all anti-inflammatory. Quercitin, 75-200 mg; and rutin, 75-150 mg included in the mix is a good idea. If the inflammation is really bad, then proteolytic enzymes are a great idea. It is a good idea to get these from a nutritionist.

## Creative Visualization

Explore the feelings with amazement and wonder of a spontaneous vacation, a distant friend knocking at your door, or a sudden insight from the divine.

## Emotional Strategies

Allow yourself to feel hopeful because even dramatic lifestyle changes can be slow in changing symptoms. Tissues take time to heal and to respond. Decide and focus on other positive emotions you want to feel.

## Relationship strategies

Set boundaries and be willing to say no. Take responsibility for your own actions and not for the actions and emotions of others. If you don't set boundaries, you are giving yourself away. This leads to resentment, burnout, and blame. You cannot be your authentic self without boundaries.

## Environmental Strategies

Limit over-the-counter medications often related to sudden bleeding from thinned blood or gastric bleeding. Acetaminophen is associated with sudden death from liver failure.

## Mental Strategies

Humor adds spontaneity and joy to life. Find out what tickles your funny bone. Is it listening to a comedian or watching a funny movie? Can you learn to tell a joke, or do you prefer to read a funny book or watch funny videos? Laughter reduces the stress responses, strengthens social connections, and releases endorphins, the feel-good hormones. It also decreases anger and can help you shift perspectives.

Remember the words of Victor Frankl, author and holocaust survivor, "Everything can be taken from a man but one thing: the last of the human freedoms—to choose one's attitude in any given set of circumstances, to choose one's own way."

## Physical Strategies

Laughter yoga is an effective way to incorporate more laughter into life, even if you don't feel like laughing. Developed by Dr. Madan Kataria, laughter yoga combines yoga breath and laughter and is a well-being workout. Laughter as a workout oxygenates the tissues, lowers blood pressure, and strengthens immunity. The body and brain cannot tell the difference between fake and real laughter so, even if you fake it, the benefits are still there. Besides that, laughter is contagious. You may not feel like laughing when you start, but you will continue giggling at the end.

## Genetic Strategies

So how do you keep your brain cells excited? What do you do to keep activating your spontaneity and your originality? Can you act on impulse and go with the flow?

High ideals, high creativity, truth and liberty, and becoming a symbol of equilibrium are ways that can express the energy of Uranus in a healthy and positive way. This means a person might be an advocate for human rights, become an architect and design energy-efficient homes, grow her own organic foods, or write an article about personal freedom. Express your unique individuality.

## CHAPTER EIGHT
# EARTH ARCHETYPES

## Earth

Earth provides the deep rich soil to grow vegetation and support life. This soil is made up of layers and layers of rock, minerals, and decaying vegetation. The dirt itself is teaming with life in the form of insects, fungus, bacteria, and more. These life forms work with plants and trees to communicate with others and mulch dying and decayed fauna and flora. This mulching process sustains the life and richness of the soil.

Many layers of the earth are solid, but the center is a hot, compressed region called the inner and outer core. The outer core is liquid, hot melted rock, which occasionally rises to the surface in volcanos. Scientists believe the very center is hot and solid due to the immense pressure exerted upon it.

The two most-common elements in the earth's crust are oxygen (46 percent) and silicon (28 percent). Because of this, the most abundant mineral in the earth's crust is silica (silicon dioxide). More commonly known as sand, silica is a major component of glass. When heated, silica melts and becomes glass, hardening as it cools. Earth is a container for water and a glass is just one example.

Metal is found throughout the earth's crust. Humans discovered that metals alone were worthless but, if they added fire, they could heat, refine, and shape metals so that they could make tools and weapons and eventually machines, panels, and support beams.

The earth has also been the source of the majority of fuels we use to produce fire. We feed our bodies with what the earth provides. We are made of the same minerals and chemicals that are of the earth. We would not be here without what she endows.

Words that express the energy of earth are grounded, foundation, manifestoes, builders, stable, practical, one step at a time, and grounding dreams into reality. Out of balance earth energy is stuck, resistant to change, stubborn, stagnant, and losing sight of spirit and emotion.

## VENUS OF TAURUS:

## HOME AND SECURITY, RELATIONSHIPS, SOUL AND CONSCIOUSNESS

### Associated Body Parts

throat

### Associated Symptoms and Diseases

any throat condition
gluttony

Robert Frost's proverb, "Good fences make good neighbors," has been around for centuries in different forms. Benjamin Franklin's version can be found in *Poor Richard's Almanac*: "Love your neighbor; yet don't pull down your hedge."

I grew up in the time of the TV show, *Bonanza*, a series about the adventures of a father and his three sons, and how they protected their home and their ranch. The land, cattle, and material possessions were sources of pride, representing their wealth and what was most valuable. They were always searching out cattle rustlers or protecting the land from invaders who didn't respect their borders. They dressed up in their string ties to go to church, socials, or community dances, and they were the "big men," the ones who had the most land and possessions.

The middle son, Hoss, a large man, played by actor Dan Blocker, had a large appetite and was comfortable in his large body. Sometimes he acted like a bumbling fool, yet he was a likable character, loved by the entire community. Each of the cast members, the father, played by Lorne Greene; the oldest son Adam, played by Pernell Roberts; and the youngest brother, played by Michael Landon, were superior "cowboys" excellent at roping, moving cattle, and training horses. It was expected of them to be good at their trade.

The home was decorated in typical Western folk art. They were at home at the ranch, with the community of workers around, and would do anything to protect their property. They were also important members of the community-at-large and helped to protect and defend the local town and its inhabitants.

This old TV show is a description of the feeling of Venus of Taurus. The feeling of those who take pride in their land and their fences. People who are good at what they do and take pride in their work, their possessions, their money, and what they produce, like farmers who take pride in their land, their crops, and can usually repair what needs repairing on the farm. They enjoy good home cooking eaten around the kitchen table, the heart of the home, and are often active members in their communities. They are not interested in fancy, just functional and practical. They have a strong desire for safety, stability, and are the salt of the earth.

The ancient world cities give rise to the same feeling and influence. This is the heritage for many of us. Walled cities throughout the world were built by nobles and landowners to protect their material possessions from invaders. The cities were filled with crafts people of all kinds: weavers, bakers, butchers, silversmiths, blacksmiths, and coopers. They lived in these walled cities for safety and security.

In Europe, the cathedral was at the center of the city. The church set the rules of behavior expected by the populace. Feast days brought the people together for singing, dancing, and the celebration of the abundance of food when harvests were plentiful and for solace when the harvest were not as abundant. They strengthened their borders when food was scarce or in the event of illness or plague.

The land still belonged to the nobleman, and it was his responsibility to protect and defend his city, his material possessions, and the people, with walls and with troops. The job included building alliances and protecting from invasion.

It is a wonderful thing to be at home in your community, also wonderful to be at home with your things about you; however I learned long ago how fleeting material possessions can be. In one night, all can be gone.

The central thing—the more vital imperative—is to be at home in your own body. To embrace your soul and consciousness for the gift that it is. Your soul, and consciousness are the only true constant. You are not your body, yet your body is there for you as a tool and vehicle to experience this world and to perceive its gifts.

Trust in your own self and your own consciousness and the wall of protection provided by the body. This is the only wall you need put around yourself, if you are at home in your body, soul, and consciousness.

It is fine to desire nice things and surround yourself with them. I love my comfortable furniture, the art on the walls, and the warm, running water. It is okay to enjoy creature comforts, yet stuff is just stuff. When being possessed by material possessions, greed, gluttony, or a rigid way of life becomes the driving force, this is the imbalance of Venus of Taurus.

Silas Marner was a weaver and an outsider to the community, because he wasn't born and raised in the town of Raveloe in the book by George Eliot. Silas had strange mannerisms and cataplectic tics, which made him appear very different. He ended up in Raveloe because he had been falsely accused of stealing, and excommunicated from the church and community to whom he belonged.

He finds nothing in the new community to interest him, and his only attempt at neighborliness backfires, so he retreats into his work, becoming a miser and a hoarder. His entire focus became his work and saving money, expanding his material wealth by collecting gold. For fifteen years he saved. At night he pulled the saved gold out from under the floorboards and counted it.

As the story unfolds, Silas has his gold stolen by the son of a squire, though Silas is unaware of who stole the money. Silas is lost and devastated. He goes to the local tavern to seek help, but no one knows who took the money, and he was told it was likely someone traveling through.

The squire's other son is secretly married to an opium addict, and they have a daughter. This son is in love with another woman, regretting the marriage and ignoring the woman and his child. One night, the secret wife heads to the squire's manor, toddler in arms, to reveal the marriage. She gets tired and stops to take some opium and falls asleep in the elements. The toddler, following the light to the nearest house, enters Silas's home. He doesn't see her because he is having one of his strange fits.

When he comes out of the fit, he finds the girl, and is first surprised and then shocked. He follows the girl's footsteps in the snow to discover that the mother is dead. He returns to the child and takes her to the squire's manor where a party is being held. He reports the death, asks for a doctor, and seeks information about the girl.

The father of the girl, who is at the party with the woman he loves, recognizes the girl and denies any knowledge of the child. He does not claim her.

Silas returns home with the child and decides to adopt her.

The community eventually begins to see Silas as a good man as he cares for the little girl, Eppie. He begins to come out of his isolation and starts to make friends. The community accepts him. Eventually he returns to church.

The story continues and has a happy resolution after many further trials, but this part of the story illustrates the message of Venus of Taurus. When Silas opened his heart to the little girl left at his doorstep, created a family and engaged in the community around him for her needs, his greed dropped away. He became happy and content in his own life and his crafting abilities. He discovered that he didn't require large amounts of material wealth to be happy and satisfied. He opened his heart to someone else and found his place within himself and in the community. A modern version of the story was retold brilliantly in a film, *A Simple Twist of Fate,* in 1994, directed by Gillies MacKinnon, with the lead played by Steve Martin.

A challenge with Venus of Taurus is having an ethnocentric worldview, when groups of people expect others to conform to a specific point of view. Religious institutions have historically set the guidelines for behavior, ostracizing and punishing those who do not conform. This type of thinking has led to fanaticism, racism, nationalism, fascism, and war. More wars have been fought over differing religions than for any other reason in the history of humankind.

Singing and the throat is related to this Venus archetype. I am reminded the German Nazi government in World War II, banning some types of music and promoting and allowing only the singing of German folk songs.

All kinds of problems continue with issues associated with fanaticism, nationalism, racism, fascism, and war in the world. In the United States, we have arguments about border walls and tremendous challenges with immigrants escaping war and tyranny. The US is not the only nation struggling with immigration problems. War and tyranny continue in multiple locations throughout the globe, leading to fear. It's really hard to be at home in your body and in your consciousness when one is living with fear. Survival and safety are the only driving forces.

The goal and task is to strengthen spiritual muscle so that one is able to choose to be at home in the body and within the beliefs that allow choosing love and compassion over fear and doubt. Strengthening kindness and benevolence within will forge new ways to bring right actions for others. Historically, people fight against what is perceived as wrong.

Build bridges of understanding rather than fearing those whose ideas, beliefs, and skin colors are different from ours. Fight for what you believe is right.

The main obstacle a person ever faces is fear. Feelings of fear are universal. Fear that one is not good enough, not healthy enough, not clever enough, are too old or too young, not resourceful enough, or not wealthy enough. There is fear about what other people will think or fear of failure. Many fear death, disability, illness.

Embracing and facing fears will enable one to walk the highest path and be authentic. Healing begins within and expands to the outside world. Be without fear as much as possible. I recall reading that the goal is to be okay with the worst thing that can happen, the primary fear. For many that fear is death. Be okay with dying. Act despite fears rather than putting up physical or emotional walls and barriers.

In addition to the throat and throat problems, Venus of Taurus issues include gluttony. Many of us have our creature comforts and too many material possessions. We also have an abundance of access to food, and it is easy to over-indulge. Over time, large quantities also lead to obesity, insulin resistance, and diabetes. Currently 42 percent of adults are obese,[44] and about one in three people are insulin resistant, meaning their cells are much less sensitive to insulin.

In a previous chapter, Venus of Libra, a male archetype, we discussed how too much sweetness and a lack of sweetness in life can be a factor in diabetes. So you can see we get a double whammy when it comes to diabetes and male and female archetypes related to Venus; overindulgence combined with a desire for more sweetness in life leads to obesity, diabetes, and all that is associated with insulin resistance. Understanding the value of what we eat, and knowing the appropriate portions, can make us more aware and prevent unintended gluttony.

## Nutritional Strategies

Macronutrients are the types of foods that we eat, versus the micronutrients, the small individual molecules that our foods break down into. Macronutrients are the foods we decide to put on our plates—the real food that provide the building blocks of our bodies. Macronutrients are the proteins, carbohydrates, and fats we get from food sources different from the vitamins and minerals, the micronutrients found in the foods.

Most people eat the same twenty foods over and over and don't experiment with different types of foods. The greater the number and types of foods, the greater the chance that you will receive an increased variety of vitamins, minerals, and the trace nutrients found in the colors of fruits and vegetables.

A teacher and mentor of mine recommends eating every color, every day. For example, broccoli is a macronutrient in the carbohydrate family. A serving of broccoli has fiber, vitamins, and phytonutrients, the nutrients from its lovely green color, and minerals when it breaks down in the digestive tract to these micronutrients. It also has pieces of proteins, amino acids, that combine with other vegetables and grains to form complete proteins.

Vegetables have parts of proteins, while animal sources provide complete proteins. People can choose to be meat eaters, vegetarians, or vegans, yet it is important for vegetarians and vegans to eat a larger variety of foods to get those complete proteins, and they may need to add a B12 supplement, because B12 is not as easily obtained in the vegetarian or vegan diet.

Proteins provide the building blocks to build, repair, and replace the tissues of the body. They break down into amino acids, which repair DNA, build enzymes, hormones, build muscles, skin, cartilage, and blood. Everyone needs a certain amount of protein to stay alive. Portions may vary depending on your body type and size but most people require about 40–60 grams/day. This is about 2–3 ounces, 2–3 times/day or servings the size of your palm without the fingers.

Fats are the foods that allow us to feel full and satiated. We need fats for every membrane of every cell in the body. Fats break down and become triglycerides, cholesterol, and essential fatty acids. Essential means that we have to eat these fats in the diet. The body cannot synthesize or create them.

The brain is 60 percent fat, so we require fat to maintain a healthy brain. Fats act as messengers, supporting proteins to do their job. We store energy with fat, and we can use fat as fuel for the brain and body. Fat also insulates and protects us.

Carbohydrates are optional for humans. We don't actually have to have them in to live, but life is better with them. They supply faster, quicker energy as they break down to blood glucose. They also spare proteins for other purposes besides energy production. Depending on the carbohydrates eaten, they regulate blood glucose. They provide flavor, and sweetness to our lives and protect our kidneys by preventing ketosis, a buildup of ketones in the body. They are sources of dietary fiber, some amino acids, phytonutrients from their multiple colors, and minerals.

Adequate sources of protein and fat can provide all the nutrients we need, especially if we eat the organ meats of animals. People who follow a ketogenic diet use fats rather than carbohydrates as their primary fuel source.

The organ meats, such as the liver, concentrate nutrients from plants so that we benefit from the B vitamins and antioxidants the animal ate while ingesting grasses and weeds. Unfortunately, like the food industry, farming has changed dramatically over the past 150 years. As noted previously, commercial animals grown in confinement are fed primarily corn and soy products rather than the wide variety of nutrients available in a healthy pasture. This has changed the quality of the protein and especially the quality of the fat in our foods.

Corn and soy are both high in omega-6 fats, which tend to be pro-inflammatory in the body. Nobody needs more inflammation! We function best when we have a balance of omega-6 fats and omega-3 fats from foods like deep ocean fish, chia seeds, flax seeds, and walnuts. It can be a challenge to get enough of these anti-inflammatory omega-3 fats in the diet. For example, farm-raised fish are also fed corn and soy so their smaller bodies concentrate the omega-6 fats. A piece of farm-raised salmon has more omega-6 fat than beef!

If you eat meat and fish, do your best to provide your body with wild-caught deep ocean fish, grass-fed beef, pastured pork or lamb, and free-range chickens. These animals are the healthiest choices having a better ratio of anti-inflammatory fats, and less likely to be raised with hormones and antibiotics.

There are many types of fats; saturated, unsaturated, mono-unsaturated, trans fats, omegas 3, 6, 9, and more. It is not important to understand everything about fats; just know to avoid fried foods and hydrogenated oils from cottonseed and soybeans. Avoid highly processed oils from corn, soy, cottonseed, or canola. Eat minimally refined, cold-pressed, oils from flax, sesame, other seeds, or avocado. Choose butter, olive oil, and coconut oils.

In addition, fat doesn't make you fat unless eaten in huge amounts. Carbohydrates make you fat because, when the body has adequate carbohydrates, it stores the excess as fat for an extra day.

Good quality fats are vital for the health of the brain and for the health of every membrane and cell in the body. Best sources are the fruits, vegetables, nuts, seeds, meats, and fish that contain fats. If you need fat to prepare foods use the least processed, minimally refined organic sources of olive, coconut, and avocado oils and real butter or ghee. Flax oil is good but should not be heated.

If you consume meat, dairy, and eggs, choose the healthiest sources that your budget will allow. Grass-fed beef, pastured pork, free-range chickens from farmers using regenerative farming practices and organic feeds are the best. Chicken and duck eggs are good sources of protein if fed with organic feed. Dairy products are good for some but not everyone. Know your farmers and their farming practices if possible.

Animal products are not necessary. Not eating them is a personal choice, which I respect; however, I can say that I have seen some mighty sick vegetarians over the years. It takes diligence and consistency to get the variety of foods to create a complete amino acid profile in the body. Amino acids are the parts of proteins that the body requires for repair and maintenance. If you just stop eating meat but continue to eat junk foods, fill up on processed grains, and skip the veggies, it is unlikely that you will feel good.

Meats are the best food source of many B vitamins, especially B12. Vegetarians often need to supplement with added B12.

If possible, know the sources of the food you eat, and know the farming practices and the farmers who raise the animals and produce that you and your family consume.

## Creative Visualization

May I take time to hear, to feel, and to reflect on my own needs and desires.
May I live in presence and awareness to expand my consciousness, and may I experience goodness in life.

## Emotional Strategies

People pleasing is seeking acceptance and love from external sources. Shift the focus to the divine feminine core to build self-love, self-acceptance, self-understanding, self-compassion, setting boundaries, and being authentic.

## Relationship Strategies

Sing together, or join a circle or group for dancing, gardening, or folk art.

## Environmental Strategies

Avoid sugar and high fructose corn syrup products as much as possible to prevent flooding the bloodstream with glucose. Over time, too much sugar leads to weight gain, insulin resistance, and diabetes. Sugar also depletes the body of needed nutrients just to digest it.

## Physical Strategies

Ask a friend or a group of friends to dance or walk with you. Having a friend makes it easier to exercise and makes it so much fun.

## Mental Strategies

Use the idea of the Big Rocks Metaphor or the strategies in Brian Tracy's book, *Eat that Frog*. The big rocks metaphor is to imagine your life as a big jar. The jar cannot be bigger because there are only so many hours in a day.

You have big rocks, small rocks, and sand. The big rocks are the most essential must do activities that make life worth living and maintain health. These vary depending on the person, but examples are working, exercising, healthy eating, and spending time with family.

The small rocks are important activities that are fun and add to fulfillment like working on a hobby, reading a good book, training for a sporting event, or working on an important or passionate project, but not as essential.

The sand is still fun but not critical for living, and you can do without, like Facebook, email, and watching television. If your day starts and continues with sand activities followed by the small rocks because it is fun and pleasurable, it leaves very little room in the jar for the big rocks. Essentials suffer, and the activities that bring health and fulfillment are put on the back burner. To-do lists continue to expand, and progress is impeded.

Time that first focuses on the big rocks followed by the small rocks, leaving the sand until last, allows the time for all the activities that bring fulfillment. "Eating the frog" means doing the most difficult tasks first to overcome procrastination and reduce anxiety. It also allows time for more fun-fulfilling activities, releasing worry about what is undone.

## Genetic Strategies

A comprehensive genetic test will indicate the right balance of proteins, carbohydrates, and fats that are appropriate for a person's optimal genetic function. These tests can also give you information about how efficient you are at processing B vitamins and if you require taking them in more activated forms. In the meantime, make those macronutrients count and enhance your vibrancy as much as possible.

Choose from the best quality products available. Visit and support your local farmer's market. These farmers work hard to provide you the best and freshest foods. The vegetables you buy at the market were likely grown organically and picked that morning. Much produce found in grocery stores is weeks or months old and has traveled cross-country or cross-continent.

## MERCURY OF VIRGO:

## CONTROL REACTIONS, RELEASE FROM OUTCOMES

### Associated Body Parts

small intestine: duodenum, jejunum, and ileum

### Associated Symptoms and Diseases

celiac disease
indigestion
bleeding
leaky gut syndrome
Crohn's disease
infections
intestinal cancer
intestinal obstruction
irritable bowel syndrome
ulcers, such as peptic ulcer

Mercury of Virgo is about control and detail, looking at the world through a microscopic lens and seeing all the tiny parts. If one has a total understanding of the tiny microscopic parts of anything it can be controlled. At least that is the illusion. The energy of Mercury in Virgo has influenced current medical treatment.

### Sick Care or Healthcare

Modern healthcare is based on the illusion of control of the body and suppression of symptoms. Medical doctors observe the body through a microscopic lens and observe the detail found in diagnostic testing. This is Western medicine as taught in university centers. Testing and imaging is utilized to try to see what is happening in an attempt to control the smallest details in the human body.

Medical doctors are trained to look at bodies, examine laboratory tests and imaging, to see what can be manipulated chemically to help a person and change a test. If the body is not broken, bleeding, or if the test is not out of range, patients are often told there is nothing wrong, even if they have symptoms. I have had so many patients over the years told by their medical doctors that their problems are all in their heads.

Training in healthcare is focused on specializing in single systems, such as cardiology, hematology, and dermatology. Often one single process or symptom is addressed by a specialist, while this same physician is unable or unwilling to look at the body as a whole. The goal is to control systems and cover symptoms with medications in hopes that the abnormal test will be manipulated to go away and in hopes that the patient will feel better and heal. The desire and plan is to control and manage the symptom often without discovering the underlying cause.

Using the strategy of powering over the disease and fighting invading organisms, the current sick-care industry is about fighting and destroying anything abnormal, often without discovering why the person is susceptible or ill in the first place.

Most medications are designed for one single little thing, one single mechanism or physiologic process in the body, yet affecting one thing is rarely possible. One small change from a medication can have a cascading effect on multiple systems and processes, resulting in a variety of effects and side effects in the person.

The family doctor of old could have been the only physician the person saw in an entire lifetime. The doctor knew the person, knew the family, knew the community and the environment. There was trust and confidence in this relationship because the patient felt understood as a whole person. The doctor who lived and worked in the same community was much more aware of the emotional and environmental factors that impacted health in the community and addressed those issues prior to prescribing any or more medication.

The medical system has moved away from this model by necessity. Family practice physicians rarely see a person for more than 10–15 minutes, just long enough to prescribe a medication or two as a trial, or to decide if there is a need to see a specialist. Much of the time the practitioner is staring at the computer screen, while in the room. So much focus in the current model is to be compliant with healthcare regulations and to have every bit of the patient encounter documented on the computer for all to access. This leaves minimal time to have meaningful conversations where patients feel heard. A patient barely has time to report symptoms, let alone share any contributing factors, before the practitioner is out the door.

Doctors hired by large medical corporations are pushed to cram as many patients as they can into their daily schedule. Most often, primary care is a nurse practitioner or physician's assistant. If the problem cannot be handled in just a few minutes, a person is sent to the specialist or multiple specialists. A specialist's job is to focus on just one area of the body, or one system, rather than looking at the body as a whole.

I recognize that medical doctors, nurse practitioners, physicians' assistants, nurses, and most all people in healthcare truly do care deeply for patients. They do the very best they can with the tools available. There is no place I'd rather be than in a trauma center in a hospital if I was injured in an accident or in the midst of a stroke or heart attack.

However, practitioners are often frustrated, restrained, and restricted by mandates from licensing boards, insurance companies, corporate healthcare, government agencies, and the pharmaceutical industry. If practitioners recommend any other care; alternative, holistic, or spiritual, it won't follow industry guidelines.

Patients too are frustrated, angry, and don't feel heard. I hear complaints daily when communicating with patients. I hear, "All they ever do is give me another pill," or "The doctor didn't listen to me," or "Nobody ever tells me what my tests mean."

Often the patients are fearful that they won't feel better or that the tests will show some devastating illness. Doctors are frequently fearful that they will do something wrong, and the patient will file a liability claim, or Medicare will discover a mistake and fine them thousands of dollars.

The sick-care industry primarily has drugs and surgery to address health conditions. This myopic way of treating people doesn't address the ways individuals are integrated and complete.

The opposite approach is to look at the big picture. One can observe the big picture and see the connections even by looking at the small, not unlike a hologram. Look at atoms under an electron microscope, and then look up to the heavens, the atoms and the galaxies above mirror each other.

We see mirrors and reflections all around, evidence of how everything is connected.

Once I was diving at Grand Cayman in the Caribbean along the beautiful deep reef found there. My first experience diving in such clear waters was glorious, seeing the neon schools of fish and the abundant sea life. I was fascinated by the black coral growing on the wall of the reef. With awe and wonder, I observed this black coral as a miniature reflection of gigantic oak trees, bare against the cold midwestern winter sky I had left at home in Iowa.

In moments of complete mindfulness and observation, I know deep within myself that this world is connected to the highest order. These connections are reflected in our human forms. There is profound beauty in the structures, the patterns, and the functions of the human body.

I attempt to see the big picture when I work with individuals. I ask questions about lifestyle and emotional and stressful situations the person may be experiencing. I observe words used and then observe the symptoms expressed by the individual. I ask the patient to use their intuition and tell me what they perceive is causing their problems.

Often the person knows and shares that there are emotional or relationship factors impacting their health. I often suggest that they use their faith, whatever faith or spiritual belief they have, to enhance their trust in the healing power of the body or to be more mindful and appreciative of the healing power of the body. When we keep the big picture in mind, it is possible to look at the smaller details, see their interconnections, and use that information to address the health challenges.

The future of healthcare will see an increased use of energy healing, more Neptune energy and feelings of interconnectedness. We are so much more powerful that we are aware of, and I see in the years ahead more and more people will tap into greater human potential, and move energy, and shift the function of cells and tissues in the body simply with energy. Just like the earth itself has an energetic electromagnetic field around it, each person is electromagnetic and has an energy field that extends well beyond the physical body.

In my years working with patients, I have learned how to measure the size of that energy field. The average size is about two to three feet out from the body. Some people's energy extends four or five feet, and some people can enter a space and fill the room with their energy.

Most people are aware when someone is in their space. When someone gets too close, it can be uncomfortable unless you have energetically invited them in by shaking hands or opening your arms for a hug. I have noticed that some people are truly oblivious to others' space. In other countries, typical distances between people vary. I have measured changes in energy fields that expand when the person has a positive thought, or has fresh organic produce near them; and shrink when asked to simply frown, or when sugar or junk food is in their energy field.

We are already seeing the use of energy healers in hospital centers now. I know of Reiki practitioners working in hospitals in New York City and medical intuitives and healing hands practitioners participating in care in a number of locations.

It is possible to move and shift energy within your own body to stimulate health and well-being. Humans experience spontaneous healing every day. Know that you can do the same.

I keep hearing of new technologies and new machines that will revolutionize healthcare in the future. Embrace the possibility that you are the technology! Upgrade your thoughts, and trust in healing. Do you need to give your power over to a machine or a handful of drugs, perpetuating a patriarchal codependent cycle?

## Digestive Issues

Daniel, age thirty-four, owned a landscaping business with a friend. He came to see me for the irritable bowel that resulted in chronic diarrhea. He was taking medications that were costing him more than $300 per month, which was a huge expense for his independent business. The meds helped a little, but he would still have episodes where he had to quickly run and find a restroom, a real challenge with his outdoor work.

In the course of our treatment program, Daniel's partner, Mitch, came up in conversation. Daniel was frustrated with Mitch, feeling like he was having to run the business alone, because Mitch was unreliable and left all the control of the business to Daniel. Daniel was resentful and angry and felt alone and out of control of the situation. He was trying to decide if he should dissolve the partnership.

A few weeks later, Daniel's condition really started turning around. He was taking some specific prescribed nutrients and had just completed a whole-body detoxification protocol following a modified elimination diet that eliminated sugars, wheat, dairy, and processed foods, and drinking nutrition shakes that focused on healing the digestive tract lining.

In addition, he told me that he and his partner chose to go separate ways. Daniel was able to buy out his partner and was running the business on his own.

Optimally, people discern what is within personal control, and what is not, and decide what allows order without being controlling. Control is an illusion. No one can control the events or the people around them though many try. Some can powerfully influence others with words or actions, yet one only has control over reactions to events or people in life. Daniel's condition stabilized and healed as he learned and healed his relationship with control. The harder he tried to control his partner, the more acute his condition became.

Persons who have issues with the energy of this archetype have challenges with a need to feel control. People who have a lot of digestive issues often feel out of control. They really want control in their world and can't have it. Besides Pluto, perfectionism can be a debilitating factor for those with Mercury in Virgo problems. The more they try to control the environment, the less control they have. Then the body begins to help, taking over what they can't control. And the symptoms begin. Bloating, indigestion, abdominal pain, and diarrhea begin. If chronic, combined with stress, it will cause irritation and destruction of the gut lining.

That's the very nature of the digestive tract. It takes in information, sorts it, decides what to take in, and it decides what is waste.

People who are strongly influenced by Mercury of Virgo can be critical, meticulous, skeptical, detail-oriented, and data-driven. They love order and compliance. Researchers, medical doctors, accountants, engineers, computer programmers, and personal assistants who do their jobs well are examples of people expressing the energy of this archetype. Our society requires their skills and abilities.

These are the people who thrive on and love order and specificity. They want the double-blind, placebo-controlled study. They need the documentation and the facts of things.

People who are detail-oriented have skills that run business, healthcare, and industry. However, they can easily get stuck in perfectionism. Imbalanced energy here can manifest with attempts to control, and being suspicious, cynical, pedantic, and small-minded. Anyone strongly influenced by this archetype doesn't want to have things change very quickly and doesn't like change for the sake of change.

A desire to have everything just perfect can be a driving force of imbalance in Mercury of Virgo. Unfortunately, this is where the downfall occurs. We can't accept "good enough." We strive to make things just right. It is easy to get stuck in inaction or anxiety. This leads to internal pressure, worry, and irritability. Often things are left unfinished due to performance anxiety.

To figure out how to make things more perfect, more organized, we recruit the digestive system to help. The organs that are associated with Virgo energy are the digestive tract and the left brain. Every receptor site that you find in the brain is also found around your gut. Your brain and your digestive tract are intimately connected. I have heard from multiple instructors over the years that "the brain is a gut and the gut is a brain."

This is a protective mechanism since the inside of the digestive tract lining is actually outside the body. A full 60 percent of the immune system sits around the digestive tract in the gut associated lymphatic tissue, known as the GALT. These brain and immune receptors are designed to protect us from absorbing things that we shouldn't and attack things that have the potential to harm us. So it is a control mechanism, deciding for us what should be absorbed and what should just pass through.

## Nutritional Strategies

The digestive tract is the system that breaks things into tiny pieces, all the way to the molecular level. In the small intestine, we find the tiny pieces of foods and where the sorting occurs.

Carbohydrates begin to break down in the mouth, and the stomach with its acids breaks all the food into smaller pieces. The small intestine continues the process. The bile from the liver/gallbladder is added to the mix in the small intestine to emulsify, break down the fats like soap. The pancreatic enzymes break apart the proteins into amino acid molecules.

Everything is designed to be broken into tiny, single or double molecule sizes. The intelligent small intestine decides which nutrients to absorb and what is to be released as waste. It controls so much! When we are stuck in detail and perfectionism, we recruit the digestive tract to step in to help us sort through issues, conflicts, decisions, and what we need to let go of.

Left long enough, we are bogged down. We can no longer sort and are unable to absorb anything. We can no longer take in anything else. The physical result is life inaction and body inaction. Foods rush through, and we can't absorb one thing more, resulting in diarrhea and an irritated digestive tract.

## Creative Visualization

Start with the end in mind. See a project or a conflict completed and resolved. The brain cannot tell the difference between something vividly and emotionally imagined and an actual experience.

## Emotional Strategies

Expand your feeling of control internally by choosing how to react to external events and emotions. Body scan mindfulness meditation may help with relaxation and awareness of different body sensations. Chant with a mantra of non-English words to take away emotion.

## Relationship Strategies

Practice a difficult conversation in your imagination first. It will give you a sense of control and confidence. Then try the conversation in person.

## Environmental Strategies

Avoid foods with artificial sugars like acesulfame K (brand names: Sunett and Sweet One), Advantame, Aspartame (two brand names: Equal and Nutrasweet), Neotame (brand name: Newtame), Saccharin (two brand names: Sweet 'N Low and Sweet Twin), Sucralose (brand name: Splenda). These products are not good for the brain and don't help with weight loss.

## Physical Strategies

Sound healing can be helpful to balance and find harmony in the external body while craniosacral therapy helps to balance the autonomic nervous system so it helps the internal body.

## Mental Strategies

Examine "should." What obligations, duties, or correctness, typically when criticizing someone's actions, do you expect?

## Genetic Strategy

One strategy to overcome the issues related is to control what needs to be controlled and be able to let go of the rest. Easy to say, but often hard to do.

The only thing we have control of is our reaction to the world around us. Take actions and learn to trust. Trust that the body knows more than the psyche and can digest food with ease. No one has to think about sending enzymes to the digestive tract or sending minerals to muscles. The body knows what to do. Trust the body, and trust that emotions can be indicators of being on the right path or that course corrections are necessary. This is epigenetics in action.

# SATURN

# REDUCING TO THE ESSENTIAL

## Associated Body Parts

bones
skin
ears
knees and other joints

## Associated Symptoms and Diseases

any chronic condition
Parkinson's
degenerative joint disease
osteopenia/osteoporosis
rickets
osteomalacia
osteogenesis imperfecta
marble bone disease (osteopetrosis)
Paget disease of bone
amyotrophic lateral sclerosis (ALS), Lou Gehrig's disease
chronic cancers
chronic heart conditions
COPD
Charcot-Marie-tooth disease (CMT)
cystic fibrosis
Ehlers-Danlos syndrome
scleroderma
fibrous dysplasia
hearing loss
psoriasis

Bernice totters into the office wearing her beige winter jacket, headscarf, and clutching a black leather handbag. She removes the flowery polyester scarf to reveal her short mousy gray hair that was obviously just washed and curled. She pats her head to make sure the hair is laying down right. It is lacquered to her head with spray to hold the hairdo until her next weekly visit to the hairdresser. She wears black polyester pants with a black-and-white geometric design pullover sweater. I greet her and tell her I will be right with her as she shuffles along in her black-laced orthopedic shoes to the treatment room.

Bernice wears her scars like a row of military medals on her chest. She has scars on her chest from the double mastectomy, on her abdomen from the hysterectomy, and on her leg from the hip replacement. She survived the war on cancer twice. She has arthritis and heart disease, and takes her seven daily medications. One for thyroid, two for blood pressure, one diuretic, two heart pills, and of course the pain reliever for her arthritis. She carries her list of medications wherever she goes. Just in case.

Our society has many versions of Bernice. She is our mother or grandmother, or the male version, great-uncle Ben. She is an example of the archetype Saturn with all her chronic disease and infirmity. Her condition is what our society tells us should be accepted: a slow gradual decline with chronic pain and illness with aging, especially as a couple of joint-replacement surgeries are added to the health history. One can't be a sissy with aging!

The traditional disease of the Saturn archetype is osteoporosis, where the foundation of the body disintegrates over time, leaving one with collapsed or broken bones. It also is the archetype of chronic disease and aging. Saturn's theme is reduction.

When I enter the room, she has her glasses off, hearing aids out, and holds a couple of tissues in her right hand. Her face is deeply wrinkled, her eyes reflect the pain she holds, and her hands are gnarled with arthritis. She is out for the day, wearing her face powder and red lipstick.

She is here for her chronic back pain. She wants me to just fix this spot in her neck before she heads off to the church luncheon. Take a little of the ache away for a little while. Please.

It is a big day; she has two outings: coming here and going to the church for a luncheon.

Her hip aches, but she tells me that her medical doctor said she has to live with it, since her heart won't allow another surgery.

I asked her what she had been eating lately, but she ignores the question. I can tell she doesn't want to go there. I have talked to her in the past about how so much sugar and carbohydrates can make her arthritis worse. Her firm expression tells me she is going to eat her breads, cookies and desserts; nobody is going to take that pleasure away.

Bernice is eighty-two and lives alone. It has been fifteen years since her husband George died from a heart attack. She shares with me that she just heard that her daughter has breast cancer now too. I tell her how sorry I am and then proceed to give her an adjustment, taking time to rub her back a little. It is likely that the last time she was touched, except for getting her hair washed and set, was the last time she was here for a visit.

Bernice needs her pain. It is her identity. She is a survivor, and she has scars to prove it. Question her, and she is happy to tell you all about her trials and struggles. I recall on her first visit just how long it took to get her health history.

She is miserable but can't see that it can be any better, so she accepts her fate. Her outings are to doctors' appointments and to church events where she can commiserate with her friends. They share the war stories of doctors' visits, whose aches and pains are worse, recovery from surgeries, who has died, and the fear of falling.

She volunteered at the hospital until it became too difficult to walk the length of the building, but she still goes for coffee there about once a week. She might run into one of her fellow volunteers that she worked with all those years.

She has no hobbies, and her eyes are getting too bad to read for more than a few minutes. She might be able to read an article in the paper, but she stopped trying to read books.

This evening, her meal is heated in the microwave as most of them are. Last night it was leftover Chinese from her lunch out with her friend Janice a few days ago. Tonight her meal is meatloaf Lean Cuisine, with peas. She eats alone, sitting with a napkin and food balanced on her lap, half-reclined in her beige La-Z-Boy.

She's watching the five o'clock local news on NBC. She is going to try *NCIS* again before bed tonight when she has her Blue Bunny strawberry ice cream and Windmill cookies. There is nothing else on, the sitcoms are so stupid, and *NCIS* disappointed her last time with so much talk of sex and violence.

It is possible to bring beauty into this parched landscape. The desert can come alive after a scant rainfall. It will burst forth with beauty as the flowers bloom and the sun reflects off the sand and flora.

Life doesn't have to be a parched desert. Life can be full and rich from beginning to end. Don't be accepting of slow debilitating decline. It doesn't have to be a battle against the body, where one achieves medals for each of the scars.

Focusing on what is essential is the key. Aging does relate to reduction, but what is reduced?

My friend Ellen may indulge in one or two glasses of wine when eating with friends, or she will enjoy some of the oatmeal cookies that she made for the grandchildren when they last visited, but she has some nonnegotiables. Any food she buys is fresh and organic.

She doesn't eat a lot of animal products but will have some fresh free-range eggs, wild line-caught fish, or some venison or elk if one of her neighbors provides it from a hunting adventure. She packs her own snacks and salads when going out for the day or when traveling across the country if she knows good food may be scarce. She is a wonderful cook who uses a wide variety of foods. It is rare for her to eat in a restaurant, since she lives about 90 miles from a large city, and she won't eat at any of the local restaurants. They have too many processed and fried foods on the menu.

Ellen lives alone since her husband Norm died, so she might eat a few more leftovers these days; and she often has a pot of bone broth and veggie soup on the stove to fill in the gaps when she doesn't want to cook for one.

She has been involved in the slow-food movement, groups of people who promote cooking healthy foods, and she goes to the group meetings. Summertime means going to the farmer's market at least once a week. She used to garden more when Norm was alive, but now she prefers the markets.

Physical activity is just as vital for her as eating well. She spent many years as a yoga instructor, however in the past ten years, she has gradually given up teaching and shifted from a yoga practice to Tai Chi and Qi Gong. In addition, she has a daily routine on her mini trampoline.

In the spring, summer, and autumn she takes a daily two-to-three mile walk up and down the mountains that surround her home and may have an adventure on the lake in her kayak, especially when the grandchildren come to visit. She is always up for a longer hike if one of her friends wants to go.

Winter you will find Ellen cross-country skiing everyday if there is enough snow to be outdoors. She lives just a short drive to downhill skiing and often goes with friends in the winter.

Ellen shared with me about a hike with a friend where they got disoriented and lost. The friend, who is eighteen years younger, ended up having to stop from exhaustion. It was growing dark, and Ellen knew she would be much too cold trying to sleep on the mountain with no gear. The friend decided to wait until Ellen could go to find help. Ellen ended up walking more than twenty miles that day before she figured out where she was and got her friend taken care of. Other than being a bit tired, Ellen suffered no adverse effects.

Health and having a team of practitioners to give her guidance is essential to her. She gets a comprehensive blood workup once a year. She uses massage therapy and sound healing. She has a local chiropractor and one in her son's hometown who she visits whenever she is staying with the family.

At five-foot-two and 114 pounds, Ellen incorporates clean eating with some detoxification protocols and intermittent fasting a couple of times a year to keep her on track and to allow healing in her digestive system. She reports feeling clear-headed and even more energetic after being even more careful with her diet.

Ellen has worked with me and a couple of other functional medicine doctors over the years. She takes her prescribed professional quality supplements religiously. The only medication she takes is a thyroid prescription. Quite a contrast from the other seventy-six-year-old women I know.

We have been fast friends for more than two decades. I know that she works at purging any nonessential actions or physical items. I have followed her through eliminating cookbooks and saving only the healthy recipes that the whole family enjoys, and purging tons of paper that she no longer requires. She has invested in programs to help her get organized and to keep only what is essential. She wants the space to do what is most important.

She releases what no longer serves, yet she still makes time for meditation, listening to books and educational programs, as well as yardwork, and creative projects.

I look to Ellen for inspiration. I know a lot about health, but I know I can bend even my own rules sometimes. I admire her ability to follow through on her nonnegotiables.

## Nutritional Strategies

Reducing to what is most essential for you to continue to live pain-free and with grace and ease is what is necessary. Perhaps that means getting essential nutrients in the form of good food or going on a daily walk. In the Blue Zones studies, the study of regions where people have greater longevity and vitality, movement is considered a vital element. So is having a social network that empowers and enlivens you.

Low energy and chronic aches and pains are the symptoms I see most in my practice as a chiropractor and nutritionist. Taking quality nutrients that support energy production can be helpful to reduce and prevent symptoms, especially if we take a number of medications that deplete nutrients faster than they can be taken in. There is not a medication that does not deplete nutrients, and many meds have a myriad of side-effects as well. Just listen to a single drug commercial on TV, and you know what I mean.

Many of the side effects of medications can be modulated by replacing the nutrients that are being washed away by the medications. This can be accomplished without reducing the potency or efficacy of the drugs.

Most bodies are not as forgiving with junk food with age. Junk foods, such as packaged, highly processed, high-calorie, low-nutrient foods, reduce body energy because they deplete the body of vitamins and minerals and use stored energy to process the non-nutrient ingredients. I know when I eat ice cream or cookies, my arthritis will flare up.

I love what Michael Pollen says in his book, *The Omnivore's Dilemma*, "Eat real food, not too much, mostly plants."

If sugar is an essential in your life, perhaps eating less of it and savoring the sweetness more mindfully can satisfy that essential need for sweetness. How many times have you eaten a favorite food, a dessert, or a chocolate without paying attention?

I recommend eating two ounces of excellent quality dark chocolate per day for those with a sweet tooth. Be a chocolate snob! Eat chocolates made only with real sugar, avoiding high fructose corn syrup. Fructose is hard on the liver.

One or two fruits per day can achieve the same result of getting that sweetness. Unfortunately we ingest so many processed, sugary foods, that fruit loses its appeal. It is not as sweet. Take a two-week break from sugar of all kinds, and then see just how sweet an apple can be!

## Creative Visualization

Say to yourself: May I find surprise and delight in all that I create. May I express with universal intelligence working through me, the vast field of knowledge and wisdom.

## Emotional Strategies

Talk with people from your past. Pull out old diaries or journals if you have them. Reflect on where you were five, ten, fifteen years ago. Ask, "Where was I and what have I done in that time?"

Notice how much has evolved and changed in your life over that time. See if there are repetitive patterns. Acknowledge just how much you have changed, experienced, and grown. Our nervous system seems wired to perpetually desire more, do more, be more, and want more. So this helps to provide balance and perspective.

## Relationship Strategies

Practice active listening, deeply empathetic listening. The more you learn of others the more you learn about yourself.

People pleasing is seeking acceptance and love from external sources. Shift the focus to the divine feminine core to build self-love, self-acceptance, self-understanding, self-compassion, setting boundaries, and being authentic.

## Environmental Strategies

Read labels and know what you are putting near, on, or into your body. Don't refill plastic bottles or food containers, even BPA-free plastics. Use stainless steel or glass when possible.

Question additional prescription medications. The third-leading cause of death in this country is medical errors, which includes prescriptions.[45] Always ask about side effects, adverse effects, and combination effects.

## Physical Strategies

Nature walks is the best way to feel in connection with all the world has to offer.

## Mental Strategies

Finding balance might mean doing less and being more; more reflective, more connected, more grounded, more joyful, more appreciative. This ties to Saturn's earth element and feminine nature. Listening to and providing the body, mind, and spirit what it needs rather than ignoring its cries for attention.

It is okay to desire more rest. Each person must decide what is essential, what is vital for their well-being. Decide what is nonnegotiable and don't let anyone interfere with those needs and desires. These essentials could manifest as a meditation practice, a spiritual practice, dancing, yoga, Tai Chi, singing, or getting a weekly massage. It can be as simple as choosing good food and good friends.

Let the nonessential go. Decrease the clutter of stuff, of information, of bad news. Give up the conversations that focus on what is not working.

Clear and declutter your spaces. Keep only what you love. This creates an environment with only essentials, the comforts that mean the most, and provides greater appreciation and joy.

There is no need to take on the problems of others. If life has been about service to others, in a move toward essential Saturn, service to self comes first, and then the energy left can be for others.

## Genetic Strategies

Reduction and getting to the heart of what is essential for life. This is the task of the Saturn archetype. The sooner one begins, the better life is. Look at all areas of life; the spiritual, emotional, relational, chemical, physical, mental, and environmental factors that contribute to a wonderful life. Decide what is absolutely needed and where life may be simpler by releasing what no longer serves. Start now, long before life defines the essential in the form of chronic disease and infirmity.

## CHAPTER NINE
# BE YOUR OWN ADVOCATE AND DEVELOP A TEAM

Wake up to your own needs. Most people have the capability and capacity to know what is best for them if they pay attention.

Some practitioners can be quite forceful in their opinions and beliefs and can come across as intimidating or frightening to patients. Words used can be threatening and scary, pressuring patients into medications or treatments they don't want or don't understand.

Know that personal opinions and beliefs are valuable and that as a healthcare consumer each person has the right to have all recommended treatments and their effects and side effects explained. It is also a personal choice to decide what treatments to undergo or to utilize.

Part of the way to be your own advocate in healthcare is to know options, look at alternatives, get more than one opinion, and make sure you choose another to be your advocate if unconscious or feel that you are not in charge of your own health.

No one should have to go to a hospital by themselves. Society is learning this from the years with COVID-19, where so many died alone, and hospital workers were overburdened and overwhelmed.

The reason the chapter on the essential is prior to this one is to decide first what is essential to happiness, fulfillment, and health, then to put the team together. Many of the players are likely in place. Most people have a primary care provider and/or a dentist. Each person needs a number of helpers, an entire team, to support them and to support good health and emotional well-being.

The best friend who understands your heartfelt desires is as important, or more important for the healthcare team as the medical doctor seen once or twice a year for a check. The medical doctor may be gone before the next visit; but your friend, no matter where they live, is only a phone call away. The friend cannot make the health decisions, but can be a listening ear to help flush out options.

A spouse or significant other is an obvious member of the team if the spouse shares similar healthcare values. If that significant person is not really a part of the healthcare team, if they don't care about health, have the same health values, or really don't understand your health needs, it is vital to have written directives in case of emergency. My spouse is also my best friend, so he will be appointed my advocate if I am ever unconscious having surgery, and he knows my wishes.

Who in your life knows your wishes and would carry them out? This can be another relative or close friend.

A team should consist of those most trusted to give the best information, the best care, and those who challenge you to be your best self.

Keep a record in your memory or on a list of the kinds of healthcare and lifestyle strategies that have had the biggest impact over your lifetime. If you walk away from a treatment feeling lighter, freer, brighter, and have less pain, then that treatment then that strategy is for you. If you feel heard, or you have an intuitive sense that this is the right choice of treatment or therapy, take note of that healing modality or that practitioner.

Symptoms don't often come on immediately, and treatments don't always have immediate results, so pay attention to feelings. Does the space where you go, the energy of the place, and the practitioner offer a good plan along with a sense of hope and possibility? If the treatment plan makes sense, then continue with the plan until it is complete.

Feeling some anxiety and fear when going to a new practitioner is normal. Health conditions often spark fear and have us imagining the worst possible outcome. It helps to go armed with a list of the symptoms you are having and the questions that require answers. When in the office, it is easy to forget the questions, so a list is valuable. The staff or practitioners may or may not appreciate the list, but that is okay. The questions and their answers are important.

Many feel intimidated by doctors because they don't understand the words used to describe the body, or they experience fear and anxiety from prior experiences. If experiencing a serious condition or have lots of questions, a second set of ears may provide a clearer picture. This is where taking a friend or a spouse along as a supportive advocate and extra set of ears to the appointment can be useful. Each person hears different things and interprets information differently. Most of us have phones that record. Turn on the recorder when the doctor enters the room, then you don't have to worry about missing something.

If you walk into an office and feel an immediate sensation of dread, darkness, or greater fear, it is time to turn around and walk out. However, if you enter a place that feels bright and hopeful, friendly faces greet you, and you sense light and positive expectation, then stick around and see what unfolds. It is important to feel hope, possibility, and optimism when addressing healthcare situations.

Even if the prognosis is not good and the inevitable outcome is death, in the case of aggressive cancer, for example, it is still important to feel hope that you can be comforted, all that can be done is being done, and that suffering can and will be minimized. It is important to feel possibility and optimism that any transition to another phase will be as graceful, peaceful, and as pain-free as possible.

Some doctors and other practitioners may have difficult personalities, yet if there is trust that the best care possible will be provided and questions are answered, then it is okay to proceed with treatment recommendations.

If you are like me and require nurturing to feel better and to heal, reach out to someone to give what others cannot. Doctors and other practitioners don't have to be nurturers to be good at what they do.

If any practitioner is not listening or not paying attention, call them out and say, "I need you to hear me." Speak slowly and clearly to express concerns and to ask about treatment recommendations. Ask to have information repeated, ask them to use words that are easily understood, ask the practitioner to slow down and to speak more slowly.

As a doctor myself, I do understand about being distracted; the healthcare office can feel like juggling, trying to keep all the balls in the air, yet the time spent with the patient is their time. The patient is paying for the time and care and has the right to have the focus and full attention of the doctor. If a patient walks away feeling confused, unseen and unheard once, the situation may be coincidental. If it happens each visit, it's time to find another practitioner.

Don't be invisible or forgotten. If expecting a test result or a referral, and no call comes, call the office. Ask to receive a call or notification with test results, whether the test is positive or negative. If you want to talk to a person about your test findings, be very clear about that. If the information on the test results in an online format, be clear about how and where to access the information and how to get questions answered if you have them. Follow-up calls may be required especially if the information is confusing.

If you are treated by more than one doctor and have prescriptions from each, ask questions to make sure that all the medications actually work together.

If you take multiple medications, an important member of the team should be a pharmacist. Ask questions about the effects and side effects of the medications you take. Read the information that is given to you when picking up a prescription. Ask about interactions between the medications you take. If a person takes more than three medications, it is difficult to know how they all work together.

Often side effects of medications don't happen immediately. Side effects can show up months or years after beginning a medication. If a new symptom suddenly develops, and there is apparently no cause, don't forget the side effects and adverse effects of medications. I cannot count how many times I have looked up a medication for a patient and found their symptom listed among the side effects of one of their drugs.

Once again, look to the areas of conflict and challenges to help see options to feeling good. The types of helpers, team members, and providers address all aspects of well-being and can result in the reduction of all kinds of symptoms.

Expect miracles and spontaneous resolution of diseases and symptoms! Miracles happen all the time! I invite those who are struggling with really debilitating conditions to search out uplifting stories of spontaneous healing, and explore the journeys these people took on the road to well-being.

A coach specializing in your career or field of study may help to find a clear path to self-growth. A new teacher in a fresh course may fuel something within. A mastermind group can be important team players, a group of individuals who come together to support each other, clarify goals and dreams, and inspire each other to take the actions that move one to bring dreams into reality. A great book discussion group can feed an internal hunger.

Structures require any or all the following practitioners: dentists, chiropractors, physical therapists, occupational therapists, personal trainers, massage therapists, and more. A myriad of modalities can stimulate healing in body tissue, and it is usually a trained practitioner who uses these modalities. Physical symptoms not resolved by other treatments may benefit from the evaluation of medical doctors, osteopathic physicians, nurse practitioners, physician assistants, naturopaths, or functional medicine specialists.

Environmental problems may require a functional medicine doctor or practitioner who can recommend and provide support in getting rid of environmental toxins or heavy metals in safe and effective ways. These support people don't have to be medical doctors but should have the training required to know what to do and how to do it. I have seen many people order products from infomercials on the internet, resulting in adverse responses and major gut problems. I know there are some great people who offer services online, however please talk to a real person, and don't buy a one-size-fits-all product because it sounds like a good idea.

Relationship support often requires a counselor or a coach who specializes in this area as part of your team. Sometimes a minister or other spiritual leader has been trained to work with couples sorting through difficult issues. If there are early childhood traumas, you will want to work with a therapist or coach who has training to work through these issues.

Emotionally, a massage therapist, a great stylist, and a nail artist may be vital to feel good. Don't forget about these service people who make a difference in people's lives. This is the area where intimate friends and some family members have their place on the team. Each person needs someone with whom they share their intimate selves. Hire a therapist or coach if there are emotional issues that require support.

Spiritually, some find their solace, and connection by belonging to a religious institution, while others feel their greatest connection and spiritual meaning walking in nature. Human beings are energy and vibration in physical bodies. Many clear up health challenges working with healers like Reiki practitioners, shamans, sound healers, medical intuitives, healing hands practitioners, and other practitioners of energy healing. These modalities can be powerful medicines and profound healing can occur. Often people feel a greater connection to God, nature, or Universal Intelligence, or feel a more profound faith after experiences with energy healing.

The chemical support team members, such as nutritionists or diet specialists, are those who can help you discover the right foods and beverages to feel great. Team members can be local farmers who grow fresh organic foods, or chefs who teach you how to combine ingredients to make foods taste great. If there are issues and the person doesn't feel good, an expert who can recommend the right professional quality nutrients can make a huge difference. There are nutritionists, naturopaths, some chiropractors and acupuncturists, or functional medicine practitioners who can help you.

The number of practitioners who work with epigenetics, examining the genes that can be positively modified with supplements and lifestyle, are few, but the number is increasing. Look in the appendix for some references. Remember, every positive strategy undertaken and incorporated positively impacts the expression of genes.

# CHAPTER TEN
# A FINAL FABLE

## "Little Brier-Rose" by Jacob and Wilhelm Grimm

A king and queen had no children, although they wanted one very much. Then one day while the queen was sitting in her bath, a crab crept out of the water onto the ground and said, "Your wish will soon be fulfilled, and you will bring a daughter into the world." And that is what happened.

The king was so happy about the birth of the princess that he held a great celebration. He also invited the fairies who lived in his kingdom, but because he had only twelve golden plates, one had to be left out, for there were thirteen of them.

The fairies came to the celebration and, as it was ending, they presented the child with gifts. The one promised her virtue, the second one gave beauty, and so on, each one offering something desirable and magnificent. The eleventh fairy had just presented her gift when the thirteenth fairy walked in. She was very angry that she had not been invited and cried out, "Because you did not invite me, I tell you that in her fifteenth year, your daughter will prick herself with a spindle and fall over dead."

The parents were horrified, but the twelfth fairy, who had not yet offered her wish, said, "It shall not be her death. She will only fall into a hundred-year sleep."

The king, hoping to rescue his dear child, issued an order that all spindles in the entire kingdom should be destroyed.

The princess grew and became a miracle of beauty, both inner and outer. One day, when she had just reached her fifteenth year, the king and queen went away, leaving her all alone in the castle. She walked from room to room, following her heart's desire.

Finally she came to an old tower. A narrow stairway led up to it. Being curious, she climbed up until she came to a small door with a small yellow key in the lock. She turned it, and the door sprang open. She found herself in a small room where an old woman sat, spinning flax. The princess was attracted to the old woman and joked with her, and said that she too would like to try her hand at spinning. She picked up the spindle, but no sooner did she touch it, than she pricked herself with it and fell down and into a deep sleep.

At that same moment, the king and his attendants returned, and everyone began to fall asleep: the horses in the stalls, the pigeons on the roof, the dogs in the courtyard, the flies on the walls. Even the fire on the hearth flickered, stopped moving, and fell asleep. The roast stopped sizzling. The cook let go of the kitchen boy, whose hair he was about to pull. The maid dropped the chicken that she was plucking. They all slept. And a thorn hedge grew up around the entire castle, growing higher and higher, until nothing at all could be seen of it.

Princes, who had heard about the beautiful Brier-Rose, came and tried to free her, but they could not penetrate the hedge. It was as if the thorns were firmly attached to their hands. The princes became stuck in them, and they died miserably. And thus it continued for many long years.

Then one day a prince was traveling through the land. An old man told him about the belief that there was a castle behind the thorn hedge, with a wonderfully beautiful princess asleep inside with all her attendants. His grandfather had told him that many princes had tried to penetrate the hedge, but that they had gotten stuck in the thorns and were pricked to death.

"I'm not afraid of that," said the prince. "I shall penetrate the hedge and free the beautiful Brier-Rose."

He went forth, but when he came to the thorn hedge, it turned into flowers. They separated, and he walked through; but after he passed, they turned back into thorns. He went into the castle. Horses and colorful hunting dogs were asleep in the courtyard. Pigeons, with their little heads stuck under their wings, were sitting on the roof. As he walked inside, the flies on the wall, the fire in the kitchen, the cook, and the maid were all asleep. He walked further. All the attendants were asleep; and still further, the king and the queen. It was so quiet, he could hear his own breath.

Finally he came to the old tower where Brier-Rose lay asleep. The prince was so amazed at her beauty that he bent over and kissed her. At that moment she awoke, and with her the king and queen, all the attendants, the horses and the dogs, the pigeons on the roof, and the flies on the walls. The fire stood up and flickered, and then finished cooking the food. The roast sizzled away. The cook boxed the kitchen boy's ears. And the maid finished plucking the chicken. Then the prince and Brier-Rose got married, and they lived long and happily until they died.

―

"Sleeping Beauty" is a tale most everyone knows from the Disney movie version. Little Brier-Rose by Jacob and Wilhelm Grimm in 1857, La Belle au Bois Dormant by Charles Perrault in the seventeenth century, and a version by Giambattisti Basile in 1634 called, "Sun, Moon, and Talia," are all retellings of a same basic tale. Some suggest the tale was carried from even earlier origins, perhaps even before the thirteenth century Icelandic legends.

This story is a metaphor for much of what I have been attempting to convey in this book. Briar Rose, the victim of a curse, is not allowed to weave her own fate, because the spinning wheels are removed or locked away. She spent most of her life sleeping, living in a coma, behind a thorny hedge, and yet she is the one who holds all the gifts bestowed on her by the fairies.

At a celebration dinner with twelve golden plates for the invited fairy guests who gift Briar Rose with everything magnificent, the thirteenth fairy arrives with the curse.

Perhaps it is a story of a father with a desire to keep his little girl young and not allow her to grow up to become a woman. Pricking her finger on the spinning wheel perhaps represents the first blood or the first menstrual cycle for the young girl. The twelve golden plates represent twelve full moons and the thirteenth moon held a curse.

But the king and queen have left out the thirteenth fairy, just as the thirteenth moon was left out of the solar calendar. Thirteen is often considered an unlucky number; and while I was growing up, I often heard that a woman's period was "the curse" and not to be spoken about . . . . So the thirteenth fairy not being invited is a lot like women not being invited to the table of men. Because there are only twelve plates (the solar/masculine year), the thirteenth fairy (the lunar/feminine year) cannot attend. Yet the thirteenth fairy shows up anyway and curses the girl. She will prick her finger; she will have her first menses. But is it a curse . . . or a blessing?

Many live life as a curse, not just cursing bodily functions like menstrual cycles and headaches, but cursing yet accepting their aches and pains, unhappiness, and frustrations as victims. Even upbeat, positive people, who I see as enlightened in many ways, still use disparaging words and sound like victims when referring to their aches and pains. Throughout history, women were obviously not invited to the table of men.

Even the men who came in search of the famed beauty and her rare gifts, a representative of the divine feminine, got stuck in the thorny hedge, because the time was not yet right for her gifts to be discovered. Only now is the divine feminine emerging in society.

The metaphor of Briar Rose is an incentive for changing what can be changed, waking ourselves out of dreams and illusions, spinning our own fate, and weaving the tapestry of our lives. The tale invites finding true love and true health within, instead of waiting to be saved by something or someone outside of us. It is accepting all the gifts that life has bestowed upon us. My invitation to you is to accept all the gifts life has bestowed upon you.

Masculine and feminine merge within this story. The thorny hedge overgrowing the castle in the story symbolizes the unknown, the darkness that bursts forth in colorful blooms when the prince goes in search of the princess. He is searching for something within, and she is awakened. The thorns represent the masculine, and the blooms the feminine, and when she awakens into full womanhood she blends the two. In the "Sun, Moon, and Talia" version, the princess gives birth to two children, Sun and Moon. Historically, the sun has been considered masculine, and the moon feminine, so she gives birth to both.

Take a moment now and celebrate the magic of the communication that is carried by the physical body. The body has input from multiple senses. Feel the messages flowing through nerves and molecules in blood to individual tissues and cells. It is truly miraculous, and the messages keep coming. Take a moment to feel gratitude and appreciation for the miracle that it is the body, and for all the ways it communicates.

Human beings are not victims of this miracle of life; and yes, each person will have symptoms. Look deep within to discover the messages, discover the causes, and to ask what is required for personal transformation. None of us will get out of here alive or completely pain-free. Listen to the messages that arise from within and take action to address what is asking for attention.

In the meantime, enjoy, appreciate, learn, and grow from the gift of all the precious moments, experiences, feelings, and relationships, and stay awake and aware as much as possible.

Look at the whole person, the physical, emotional, chemical, spiritual, mental aspects and how these multiple aspects interact with each other and in the environment and in relationships. All beings are wonderfully connected in ways that continue to unfold.

Examine the multiple strategies that can be incorporated beyond and including traditional healthcare. Know what personal essentials are required for good health and a fulfilling life, and strive to include these nonnegotiable requirements. This is self-care and self-compassion.

I heard someone on YouTube the other day ask, "When are we ever going to be done with healing?" The answer is never. Healing is a lifelong process that ends only with death. There is always something to be uncovered or to be healed and transformed. Cells in the body are turned over and replaced in a continuing process, so healing never ends. Be grateful for this automatic activity.

Wake up to personal responsibility and be a good advocate for yourself. This means eating real food and noticing how the food affects the physical body. Communication with ourselves and others can always be enhanced, and relationships can continually be improved.

Wake up to the impact of genetic expression, and trust in the ability to positively change it. Look to a future bright with knowledge about how DNA can be further enhanced with lifestyle.

Wake up to hope and possibility.

Wake up to your part in creation, and know that life is for you.

Wake up to feeling good.

# APPENDIX

## GENETIC INFORMATION

DNA testing is now relatively inexpensive. A simple cheek swab or cells found in saliva will provide a treasure of genetic data. Some companies specialize in unique heritage to search out family history. Many private companies test genetics. In my practice, I use a private company that tests many genetic markers related to brain and body function. I test for over 700 genes. Each of these genes have studies related to their function and provide valuable information on how the individual's body functions. We know that it is no one-gene-one-function, but an interplay between the genes that turn on and turn off specific processes in the body.

Some practitioners look for the genetic markers related to disease, looking for the markers to tell people what diseases one may get or drugs that may be needed in the future; while other practitioners look to epigenetic information; the genetic variants that can be positively impacted by lifestyle and nutrient changes.

Research continues to demonstrate that thoughts, movement, environment, and foods all impact genetic expression. Decide to impact genetic function positively by being optimistic, moving frequently, limiting exposure to toxins as much as possible, and eating real food, including lots of plants.

An increasing number of practitioners work with modifiable factors related to gene expression, especially utilizing nutrition and lifestyle. These lifestyle changes and specific nutrients may have significant positive impact on many genetic pathways and biochemical reactions in the body.

I have studied the genes that code for and regulate the activity of specific enzymes. Enzymes act as catalysts in living organisms regulating the rate in which biological processes occur. The enzymes affect the function of the cardiovascular, neurological, hormonal, digestive, immune, and detoxification systems in the body.

Enzymes require effective energy production, cofactors, such as specific minerals and vitamins, and a process called methylation to function correctly. "Methylation is a simple biochemical process, the transfer of four atoms—one carbon atom and three hydrogen atoms (CH3)—from one substance to another. When optimal methylation occurs, it has a significant positive impact on many biochemical reactions in the body that regulate the activity of the cardiovascular, neurological, reproductive, and detoxification systems, including those relating to: DNA production, neurotransmitter production, histamine, estrogen, and fat metabolism, detoxification, and liver and eye health.

The body is a very complex machine, with various gears and switches that need to be all functioning properly to operate optimally. Think of methylation, and the opposite action, demethylation, as the mechanism that allows the gears to turn, and turns biological switches on and off for a host of systems in the body."[46]

Seven specific nutrients can help the methylation cycle achieve optimal performance, even if an individual has the genetic mutation that slows down the methylation cycle.

1. 5-MTHF (active folate)
2. methylcobalamin (active vitamin B12)
3. pyridoxal 5'phosphate (active vitamin B6)
4. riboflavin 5'phosphate (active vitamin B2)
5. magnesium
6. betaine (AKA trimethylglycine)
7. vitamin D

Proper methylation influences so many systems in our bodies that it often gets overlooked, which can severely impact how well your body functions.

The genes are related to processes including effectively making energy, keeping inflammation reduced, improving sleep, preventing birth defects, stimulating immune function, keeping the brain happy, detoxifying through appropriate pathways, and helping in the prevention of heart disease, cancer, dementia, diabetes, and much more. To learn more about genetic testing contact myhappygenes.com and ask for a doctor to help you.

## POSITIVE STRATEGIES

Say "I don't know" if you don't know.
Take a cooking class.
Learn a new sport.
Be honest.
Stand out in a crowd.
Confess your blunders to a friend.
Say no when you mean no.
Accept a compliment.
Take a break.
Give a gift for no reason at all.
Stargaze.
Smile at a stranger.
Cultivate good friends.
Make a daily checklist.
Keep a journal.
Ask for something you want.
Share your interests with others.
Risk embarrassment.
Hire a coach.
Attend a craft fair.
Be considerate in traffic.
Forgive yourself (or another).
Speak the truth.
Brainstorm.
Listen.
Initiate a conversation.
Complete the task in front of you.
Let someone else go first.
Paint a wall
Wear something daring
Pamper yourself
Send a love note.
Hug—a lot!
Take a nature walk.
Hit a pillow.
Spend time alone.
Ask questions.
Lie on the grass.
Focus on a hobby.
Knit.
Do research on the internet.
Join a dating service.
Express gratitude daily.
Adjust your standards.
Renegotiate your agreements.
Visit a museum.
Practice the art of conversation.
Read a book.
Be interested.
Give a compliment.
Ask for help.
Meditate.
Put emotional boundaries in place.

Create something.
Take a class you put off.
Breathe.
Eat right.
Get enough sleep.
Speak so others can hear you.
Call someone who loves you.
Pet the cat.
Give yourself a positive treat.
Do something kind for someone else.
Appreciate weather/rain or shine.
Listen to music.
Take a mental vacation.
Clean the bathroom.
Watch a comedy.
Throw a dinner party.
Say you're sorry.
Stand for your convictions.
Exercise.
Get professional help.
Plant some flowers.
Sing out loud.
Dance.

Design a new business card.
Walk the dog.
Cry.
Listen to the birds.
Smell a flower.
Pray.
Flirt.
Attend a recital.
Write five affirmations.
Change your mind.
Be willing to be wrong.
Get (or give) a massage.
Eliminate silent contracts.
Take a bath.
Obtain knowledge.
Run through the sprinklers.
Focus on one thing at a time.
See another's point of view.
Check in with a friend.
Get out of your own way.
Break your own rules.
Say hello to those you encounter.
Follow your intuition.

Those of us who have held a job know the pressure of work-related stress. In fact, 65 percent of Americans cited work as a top source of stress according to the American Psychological Association. With the majority of our days spent at the office, it's important to know how to cope with everyday stressors.

It's not realistic to think you can lay out a mat and start your flow in the hallway of the office or dance like nobody's watching, because all your coworkers are. Instead, try the following relaxation techniques that you can do right at your desk!

Browse through our office-approved, stress-relief activities!*

- ❖ Go to your happy place. Sometimes it's all about visualization and tapping into all your senses. And by all, we mean all. Start by thinking of a relaxing moment in your life, when everything seemed to be at ease. Where were you? What did you see, smell, or feel? Tapping into these specific details is a great way to refocus your attention and overwhelm your body with feelings of ease.
- ❖ Try deep breathing. You might be wondering how to relax your mind. It's all about deep breathing. Concentrate on relaxing your body from your head to your toes as you inhale and exhale. This will increase the supply of oxygen to your brain and lead you into a state of calm.
- ❖ Goof off a little. Keep a stash of funny stuff somewhere near your desk, or crack a joke in the kitchen. Don't forget that laughing at yourself is a good way to stay humble and a nice reminder not to take life too seriously.
- ❖ Watch a funny video. If goofing off on your own isn't working out for you, try watching a funny video. Laughter has been shown to reduce the physical effects of stress while boosting creativity and productivity!
- ❖ Diversify your snacks. Having something to look forward to throughout the work day can help to get your mind off all the things that may be worrying you. The right snack can also give your blood sugar a boost and improve your overall energy. Think dark chocolate, blueberries, and yogurt.

- ❖ Listen to music. Create a soothing playlist for yourself, and put it on whenever you're feeling overwhelmed. Music has a unique link to our emotions and the power to relax the mind. Pick a slow and soothing soundtrack or try out a white noise playlist.
- ❖ Take a moment to gaze out of the window. If there's absolutely no way you'll be able to make a trip outside during your day, at least take a moment to gaze out of the window. Getting your mind away from the screen can actually make you more productive.
- ❖ Write yourself a positive message. Your desk is bound to be filled with notepads and a container of pens, so grab one and jot down a positive message about yourself. Try "I am the best [insert what you do]." Our brains are constantly running and there's a high percentage of our thoughts that are negative. Cancel out that negative self talk with something positive.
- ❖ Get a desk diffuser. Did you know that scents can have an impact on your stress levels? Grab a desk diffuser and try out lavender essential oils for stress relief.
- ❖ Take one thing at a time. This one is easier said than done, but it's worth the effort. Instead of thinking about all the things on your plate, grab your notepad and make a list of the tasks you'd like to accomplish today. Then focus on one thing at a time, physically cross items off your list as you accomplish them.

*Adapted from Rhonda Britten *Fearless Living: Overcome Fears & Become Your Ultimate Self* and Shari's Berries

# ENDNOTES

1. Manyema M, Norris SA, Richter LM. Stress begets stress: the association of adverse childhood experiences with psychological distress in the presence of adult life stress. BMC Public Health. 2018 Jul 5;18(1):835. Doi: 10.1186/s12889-018-5767-0. PMID: 29976168; PMCID: PMC6034311.
2. Walton DM, Tremblay P, Seo W, Elliott JM, Ghodrati M, May C, MacDermid JC. Effects of childhood trauma on pain-related distress in adults. Eur J Pain. 2021 Nov. 25(10):2166-2176. Doi: 10.1002/ejp.1830. Epub 2021 Jul 9. PMID: 34196073.
3. Archival Report| Volume 80, ISSUE 5, P372-380, September 01, 2016 Holocaust Exposure Induced Intergenerational Effects on *FKBP5* Methylation Rachel Yehuda. Published: August 12, 2015 DOI:https://doi.org/10.1016/j.biopsych.2015.08.005
4. Dr. Mary Lou Rane, NET Therapy: Key Benefits and What to Expect. https://www.drmarylourane.com/net-therapy-key-benefits-and-what-to-expect/ See also www.netmindbody.com
5. Young EH, Pan S, Yap AG, Reveles KR, Bhakta K. Polypharmacy prevalence in older adults seen in United States physician offices from 2009 to 2016. *PloS One*. 2021 Aug 3;16(8):e0255642. Doi: 10.1371/journal.pone.0255642. PMID: 34343225; PMCID: PMC8330900.
6. Varghese D, Ishida C, Haseer Koya H. Polypharmacy. [Updated 2022 May 2]. In: StatPearls [internet]. Treasure Island (FL): StatPearls Publishing; 2022 Jan. https://www.ncbi.nlm.nih.gov/books/NBK532953/
7. The Healing Power of Illness: Understanding What You Symptoms are Telling You. Ruediger Dalke, MD, Thorwald Dethlefsen et al. March 7, 2016, Pg. 7

8. Stone, Merlin. *When God Was a Woman*. New York: Barnes & Noble Book, 1993.
9. Kirsch, Jonathan. *God Against the Gods: The History of the War Between Monotheism and Polytheism*. New York: Viking Compass, 2004, 3: Stone.
10. Pagels, Elaine. *Adam, Eve, and the Serpent*. New York: Random House, 1988.
11. Almodóvar-Reteguis, Navda L. "Where in the World do Women Still Face Legal Barriers to Own and Administer Assets?" World Bank Blogs. https://blogs.worldbank.org/opendata/where-world-do-women-still-face-legal-barriers-own-and-administer-assets.
12. Warner, Marina. *Alone of All Her Sex: The Myth and the Cult of the Virgin Mary*. New York: Alfred A. Knopf, 1976.
13. Martin, Michel with Beverly Guy-Sheftall. "A Look Back at Women's Studies Since the 1970s." *Tell Me More*. National Public Radio. 17 March 2010. https://www.npr.org/templates/story/story.php?storyId=124775888
14. Gruber, Freya M., Distlberger, Eva, Scherndl, Thomas, Ortner, Tuulia M., and Pletzer, Belinda. "Psychometric Properties of the Multifaceted Gender-Related Attributes Survey (GERAS)." *European Journal Psychological Assessment*. July 2020. 36(4):612–623. doi:10.1027/1015-5759/a000528. https://pubmed.ncbi.nlm.nih.gov/32913384/
15. Chilet-Rosell, Elisa. "Gender Bias in Clinical Research, Pharmaceutical Marketing, and the Prescription of Drugs." *Global Health Action*. 9 December 2014. 7:10.3402/gha.v7.25484. doi:10:3402/gha.v7.25484. https://www.ncbi. nlm.nih.gov/pmc/articles/PMC4262757/
16. The Kybalion. Chapter XIII, "Gender." https://www.sacred-texts.com/eso/kyb/kyb15.htm
17. Denson, Thomas F., Siobhan M. O'Dean, Khandis R. Blake, and Joanne R. Beames. "Aggression in Women: Behavior, Brain, and Hormones." *Frontiers in Behavioral Neuroscience*. 2 May 2018. https://www.frontiersin.org/articles/10.3389 /fnbeh.2018.00081/full
18. Eagley, AH & Steffen, VJ. "Gender and Aggressive Behavior: A Meta-analytic Review of the Social Psychological Literature." *Psychological Bulletin* 100:3, 1986, 309-30, https://psycnet.apa.org/doi=10.1037%2F0033-2909.100.3.309; Crick, Nicki R. and Kenneth A. Dodge.

"Social Information-Processing Mechanisms in Reactive and Proactive Aggression." *Child Development*, Vol. 67, No. 3 (June 1996), 993-1002. https://srcd.onlinelibrary.wiley.com/doi/10.1111/ j.1467-8624.1996.tb01778.x).

[19] Fariha, Angum, Tahir Khan, Jasndeep Kaler, Lena Siddiqui, and Azhar Hussain. "The Prevalence of Autoimmune Disorders in Women: A Narrative Review." *Cureus,* 13 May 2020. https://www.ncbi.nlm.nih.gov/pmc/articles/PMC7292717/

[20] *Washington Post,* Outlook Section, 13 September 2019.

[21] Spencer Harvey. Glaad's Where We Are On TV Report: LGBTQ Representation On Broadcast TV Reaches Record-High, With Growing Racial Diversity And Advances In Lesbian And Transgender Representation. Feb 17, 2022
https://www.glaad.org/releases/glaad%E2%80%99s-where-we-are-tv-report-lgbtq-representation-broadcast-tv-reaches-record-high

[22] *The New York Times Magazine,* "The 1619 Project." https://www.nytimes.com/interactive/2019/08/14/magazine/1619-america-slavery.html

[23] Catherine Porter. "The Root of Haiti's Misery: Reparations to Enslavers. *The New York Times*, May 26, 2022. https://www.nytimes.com/spotlight/haiti

[24] Perez-Bret E, Altisent R, Rocafort J. Definition of compassion in healthcare: a systematic literature review. Int J Palliat Nurs. 2016 Dec 22(12):599-606. doi: 10.12968/ijpn.2016.22.12.599. PMID: 27992278).

[25] Sapolsky, Robert. *Why Zebras Don't Get Ulcers: An Updated Guide to Stress, Stress Related Diseases, and Coping (2nd Edition).* W. H. Freeman. 1998.

[26] Ford, Debbie. *The Dark Side of the Light Chasers" Reclaiming your Power, Creativity, Brilliance, and Dreams.* Riverhood Books. 2010.

[27] Williams, S.E. et al. The Power of Negative and Positive Episodic Memories. *Cognitive, Affective and Behavioral Neuroscience.* 22. Springer. 2022.

[28] Berridge MJ. Vitamin D deficiency and diabetes. *Biochem J.* 2017;474(8):1321–1332. Mar 24, 2017. doi:10.1042/BCJ20170042

29. Niaz K, Zaplatic E, Spoor J. Extensive use of monosodium glutamate: A threat to public health?. *EXCLI J*. 2018;17:273-278. Published 2018 Mar 19. doi:10.17179/excli2018-1092
30. *Heart: A History* by Sandeep Jauhar, Patrick Lawlor, et al. Picador, 2019.
31. De Strijcker D, Lapauw B, Ouwens DM, Van de Velde D, Hansen D, Petrovic M, Cuvelier C, Tonoli C, Calders P. High-Intensity Interval Training. *J Musculoskelet Neuronal Interact*. 2018 Jun 1;18(2):215-226. PMID: 29855444; PMCID: PMC6016496.NIH https://pubmed.ncbi.nlm.nih.gov/29855444/
32. Tsuzuku S, Kajioka T, Sakakibara H, Shimaoka K. Scand J Med Sci Sports. 2018 Apr;28(4):1339-1344. doi:10.1111/sms.13039. Epub 2018 Jan 30. PMID: 29247985.
33. The Extraordinary Science of Junk Food. *The New York Times*. 2.24.13. https://www.nytimes.com/2013/02/24/magazine/the-extraordinary-science-of-junk-food.html?smid=url-share
34. NIH Overweight and Obesity Statistics 2017–2018 data from the National Health and Nutrition Examination Survey (NHANES) https://www.niddk.nih.gov/health-information/health-statistics/overweight-obesity. Source: Summary Health Statistics Tables for U.S. Adults: National Health Interview Survey, 2018, Table A-4b, A-4c pdf icon[PDF – 137 KB]
35. "intermittent Fasting: What is it, and how does it work? Johns Hopkins Medicine https://www.hopkinsmedicine.org/health/wellness-and-prevention/intermittent-fasting-what-is-it-and-how-does-it-work#
36. The 1-Year Mortality of Patients Treated in a Hip Fracture Program for Elders Scott Schnell, MD, Susan M. Friedman, MD, MPH, Daniel A. Mendelson, MS, MD, Karilee W. Bingham, MS, RN, FNP, and Stephen L. Kates, MD. *Geriatr Orthop Surg Rehabil*. 2010 Sep; 1(1): 6–14.
37. See The work of Byron Katie. https://thework.com/school-for-the-work-byron-katie
38. Fowke JH, Longcope C, Hebert JR. Cancer Epidemiol Biomarkers Prev. 2000 Aug;9(8):773-9. PMID: 10952093. Kapusta-Duch J, Kopeć A, Piatkowska E, Borczak B, Leszczyńska T. Rocz Panstw Zakl Hig.2012;63(4):389-95. PMID: 23631258.

39   Ebara S. Nutritional role of folate. Congenit Anom (Kyoto). 2017 Sep; 57(5):138-141. doi: 10.1111/cga.12233. Epub 2017 Jul 25. PMID: 28603928. Valdés-Ramos R, Guadarrama-López AL, Martínez-Carrillo BE, Benítez-Arciniega AD. Vitamins and type-2 diabetes mellitus. Endocr Metab Immune Disord Drug Targets. 2015;15(1):54-63. doi: 10.2174/1871530314666141111103217. PMID: 25388747; PMCID: PMC4435229.

40   Center for Disease Control, 2010.

41   "Tipping the Sugar Scales," BambooCare. www.bamboocarefitness.com

42   Emily F. Hittner, Jacquelyn E. Stephens, and Claudia M. Haase. Positive Affect Is Associated With Less Memory Decline: Evidence from a 9-year longitudinal study. *Psychological Science*. Sage Journals. Vol 31; Issue 11. Oct 22, 2020. https://journals.sagepub.com/doi/10.1177/0956797620953883

43   "Hormones reveal the secret life of fat cells: Understanding the slew of compounds produced by fat might one day lead to therapeutics for obesity-related conditions" by Jyoti Madhusoodanan, special to C&EN, October 6, 2018 | A version of this story appeared in Volume 96, Issue 40 *Chemical and Engineering News*.

44   *Am J Respir Crit Care Med*. 2018 Feb 16. doi: 10.1164/rccm.201706-1311OC.

45   Hales CM, Carroll MD, Fryar CD, Ogden CL. Prevalence of obesity and severe obesity among adults: United States, 2017–2018. NCHS Data Brief, no 360. Hyattsville, MD: National Center for Health Statistics, 2020.

46   Roel E, García-Díez M, Borrás Bermejo B. Errores médicos, ¿la tercera causa de muerte en Estados Unidos? [Medical errors, the third leading cause of death in the United States?]. *J Healthc Qual Res*. 2019;34(6):339-341. doi:10.1016/j.jhqr.2019.06.005

47   Alan Miller, ND, What Is Methylation and Why Should We Care About It, in *Take 5 Daily*, Thorne. September 3, 2018. https://www.thorne.com/take-5-daily/article/what-is-methylation-and-why-should-you-care-about-it#:~:text=Methylation%20is%20getting%20its%20fair,molecules%20act%20in%20the%20body.

# ACKNOWLEDGMENTS

I have been so blessed to have so many wonderful people who have made this book possible.

This work would not have been possible without Rudiger Dahlke who introduced me to the planetary influences, and Carol Greenhouse who made it possible to study them.

My sincere thanks to Dawn Morningstar whose influence started this project and who helped me with the creative visualizations.

Steffany Kroeger whose help with the emotional and mental strategies was gratefully appreciated.

Mark Waldman your work is powerful and speaks for itself. I am truly grateful.

Special thanks to Dr. J. Dunn for having a conversation with me about the genetic information.

Thanks to Marly Cornell for your fantastic editing, you took a mess and made it readable. Carol Chambers for further editing and letting me know where to cut. I appreciate you.

I am so thankful to Christine Ishananda Maxwell for the beautiful cover art.

Tifanie Wells, Elizabeth Patricia Connor, Lisa Walker, and Jean Shoenecker I don't know what I would do without your love and encouragement.

Many thanks to all the patients who have given me the honor of joining them on their healing journey. I am truly grateful for your faith and confidence.

Thank you, Andrea and Karl for checking on your mother and of course Michael who supported me in so many ways.

# ABOUT THE AUTHOR

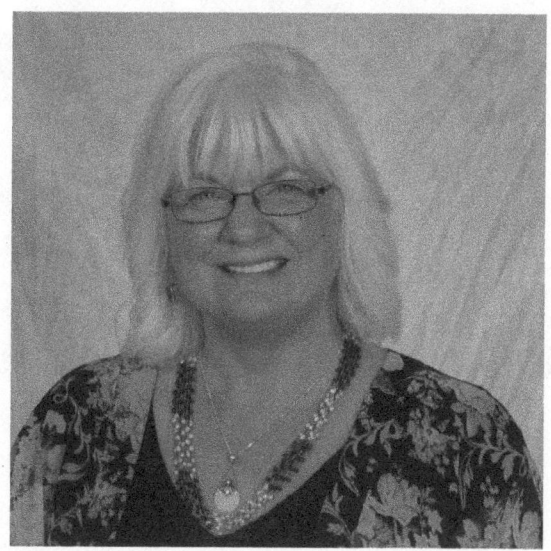

Dr. Valorie Prahl is a Doctor of Chiropractic, Certified Clinical Nutritionist, and an integrative practitioner in active practice for more than thirty-five years. Her frustration with the typical medical approach of suppressing symptoms without finding their underlying cause set her on a journey to discover solutions.

Dr. Prahl has spent decades exploring alternative healing and ways to help others. She knows that we are spiritual beings having a human experience and she understands how people get ill and how they can progress to health. Over the past several years, she has been learning and exploring ancient healing arts and energy healing practices as well as genetic optimization. The body has an innate ability to heal once the causes of disease and ill health are illuminated. www.valprahl.com